The Pediatric Cardiology Handbook

The Pediatric Cardiology Handbook

MYUNG K. PARK, M.D.
Professor of Pediatrics
Head, Division of Cardiology
The University of Texas Health Science
Center at San Antonio
San Antonio, Texas

Mosby
Year Book

St. Louis Baltimore Boston Chicago London
Philadelphia Sydney Toronto

Mosby
Year Book

Dedicated to Publishing Excellence

Sponsoring Editor: Stephanie Manning
Assistant Managing Editor, Text and Reference: Jan Gardner
Production Project Coordinator: Karen Halm
Proofroom Supervisor: Barbara Kelly

Mosby-Year Book, Inc.
11830 Westline Industrial Drive
St. Louis, MO 63146

1 2 3 4 5 6 7 8 9 0 M C 95 94 93 92 91

Library of Congress Cataloging-in-Publication Data
Park, Myung K. (Myung Kun), 1934-
The pediatric cardiology handbook/Myung K. Park.
p. cm.
Includes bibliographical references.
Includes index.
ISBN 0-8151-6612-5
1. Pediatric cardiology—Handbooks, manuals, etc. I. Title.
[DNLM: 1. Cardiovascular Diseases—in infancy & childhood—
-handbooks. WS 39 P236p] 91-13372
RJ421.P38 1991 CIP
618.92′ 12—dc20
DNLM/DLC
for Library of Congress

NOTICE

Every effort has been made to ensure that the drug dosage schedules herein are accurate and in accord with the standards accepted at the time of publication. However, as new research and experience broaden our knowledge, changes in treatment and drug therapy occur. Therefore, the reader is advised to check the product information sheet included in the package of each drug he plans to administer to be certain that changes have not been made in the recommended dose or in the contraindications. This is of particular importance in regard to new or infrequently used drugs.

Dedicated to my wife, Issun, and our boys, Douglas, Christopher, and Warren.

Preface

Many comprehensive text and reference books are available for the specialist and trainee in pediatric cardiology. New entries into the field and revisions of standard texts are appearing with greater frequency, reflecting the increasing body of knowledge of cardiovascular pathophysiology in children and the new diagnostic and therapeutic options available to the specialist. To the nonspecialist, however, these books are not always entirely useful, because they are filled with many details beyond the need or the comprehension of the practitioner of pediatric primary care or the student.

The *Pediatric Cardiology Handbook* has been written and produced to meet the needs of pediatricians, family physicians, residents, and medical students. It is intended to serve as a portable, accessible reference manual for nonspecialists in pediatric cardiology. Emphasis is on the diagnosis and nonoperative management of the more common cardiac disorders seen in children. In addition, the outline format of this handbook should further aid the nonspecialist in arriving at management decisions quickly while on rounds or in a busy office. For the inexperienced the *Pediatric Cardiology Handbook* should facilitate introduction to cardiac care in children. For the more experienced nonspecialist it should serve as a refresher for common routines, normal values, and drug dosages, and a handy guide for managing problems encountered for the first time.

This handbook is not intended to replace standard texts on pediatric cardiology; rather, it is hoped that the *Pediatric Cardiology Handbook* will be used by students, residents, and practitioners in conjunction with the major pediatrics texts and with pediatric cardiology texts when called for.

I thank Mrs. Diane Halim for her able handling of the manuscript, which required many revisions. Grateful acknowledgement also goes to Drs. John H. Calhoon, Deborah Rasch, and Da-Hae Lee for their many contributions to the handbook.

Myung K. Park, M.D.

Frequently Used Abbreviations

AR	Aortic regurgitation
AS	Aortic stenosis
ASD	Atrial septal defect
BBB	Bundle branch block
CAH	Combined atrial hypertrophy
CHD	Congenital heart disease or defect
CHF	Congestive heart failure
COA	Coarctation of the aorta
CPB	Cardiopulmonary bypass
CXR	Chest x-ray
DORV	Double-outlet right ventricle
Echo	Echocardiography or echocardiographic
HLHS	Hypoplastic left heart syndrome
HOCM	Hypertrophic obstructive cardiomyopathy
IHSS	Idiopathic hypertophic subaortic stenosis
IVC	Inferior vena cava
LA	Left atrium or left atrial
LAD	Left axis deviation
LAE	Left atrial enlargement
LAH	Left atrial hypertrophy
LBBB	Left bundle branch block
LICS	Left intercostal space
LLN	Lower limit of normal
LLSB	Lower left sternal border
LPA	Left pulmonary artery
LPL	Left precordial lead
L-R shunt	Left-to-right shunt

LRSB	Lower right sternal border
LSB	Left sternal border
LV	Left ventricle or left ventricular
LVE	Left ventricular enlargement
LVH	Left ventricular hypertrophy
LVOT	Left ventricular outflow tract
MLSB	Mid–left sternal border
MPA	Main pulmonary artery
MR	Mitral regurgitation
MRSB	Mid–right sternal border
MS	Mitral stenosis
MVP	Mitral valve prolapse
PA	Pulmonary artery or posteroanterior
PAC	Premature atrial contraction
PAPVR	Partial anomalous pulmonary venous return
PAT	Paroxysmal atrial tachycardia
PBF	Pulmonary blood flow
PDA	Patent ductus arteriosus
PR	Pulmonary regurgitation
PS	Pulmonary stenosis
PV	Pulmonary vein or pulmonary venous
PVC	Premature ventricular contraction
PVM	Pulmonary vascular markings
PVOD	Pulmonary vascular obstructive disease
PVR	Pulmonary vascular resistance
RA	Right atrium or right atrial
RAD	Right axis deviation
RAE	Right atrial enlargement
RAH	Right atrial hypertrophy
RBBB	Right bundle branch block
RICS	Right intercostal space
RPA	Right pulmonary artery
RPL	Right precordial lead
R-L shunt	Right-to-left shunt
RV	Right ventricle or right ventricular
RVE	Right ventricular enlargement
RVH	Right ventricular hypertrophy
RVOT	Right ventricular outflow tract

S1	First heart sound
S2	Second heart sound
S3	Third heart sound
S4	Fourth heart sound
SBE	Subacute bacterial endocarditis
SEM	Systolic ejection murmur
S-P shunt	Systemic-to-pulmonary shunt
SVC	Superior vena cava
SVR	Systemic vascular resistance
SVT	Supraventricular tachycardia
TAPVR	Total anomalous pulmonary venous return
TGA	Transposition of the great arteries
TOF	Tetralogy of Fallot
TR	Tricuspid regurgitation
TS	Tricuspid stenosis
ULN	Upper limit of normal
ULSB	Upper left sternal border
URSB	Upper right sternal border
VSD	Ventricular septal defect
VT	Ventricular tachycardia
WPW	Wolff-Parkinson-White (syndrome)

Contents

ROUTINE CARDIAC EVALUATION IN CHILDREN

I

I. HISTORY TAKING

Important cardiovascular histories in infants and children include the following.

A. Gestational and Perinatal History:

1. Maternal infection: Rubella (rubella syndrome: PDA, and PA stenosis). Other viral infections may be teratogenic or may cause myocarditis.
2. Medications and alcohol: Amphetamines, anticonvulsants, progesterone/estrogen are highly suspected teratogens. Alcohol may cause fetal alcohol syndrome (in which VSD, PDA, ASD, and TOF are common)..
3. Maternal illnesses: Maternal diabetes (increased incidence of CHD [TGA, VSD, and PDA], and cardiomyopathy). Lupus erythematosus or collagen diseases (congenital heart block in the offspring).

B. Postnatal and Present History:

1. Poor weight gain and delayed development (CHF, severe cyanosis, or general dysmorphic conditions).
2. Cyanosis, squatting, and "cyanotic spells" (TOF and other cyanotic CHD).
3. Tachycardia, tachypnea, and puffy eyelids are signs of CHF.
4. Frequent lower respiratory tract infections (large L–R shunt lesions).

5. Decreased exercise tolerance.
6. Heart murmur (age when first heard; association with fever?).
7. Chest pain (Related to activity? Duration, nature, radiation).
8. Palpitation (commonly caused by paroxysms of tachycardia or single premature beats).
9. Joint pain (joints involved, duration, migratory or stationary, recent sore throat, rashes, family history of rheumatic fever).
10. Neurologic symptoms: Stroke from embolization or thrombosis from polycythemia or infective endocarditis. Headache from polycythemia or hypertension (±). Choreic movement from rheumatic fever. Syncope from arrhythmias, long QT syndrome, or mitral valve prolapse.
11. Medications, cardiac and noncardiac (name, dosage, timing, duration).
12. Diseases of other systems with associated cardiovascular manifestations (Tables 1–1 and 1–2).

C. Family History:

1. Selected hereditary diseases with certain forms of CHD are listed in Table 1–1.
2. CHD in the family: The incidence of CHD in the general population is about 1% (8–12/1,000 live births). With one affected first-order relative the incidence increases by threefold (3%); with two affected members the incidence increases to 9%; with three affected family members the incidence may be as high as 50%.
3. Rheumatic fever frequently occurs in more than one member of the family.

II. PHYSICAL EXAMINATION

A. Inspection:

1. General appearance: (1) happy or cranky; (2) nutritional state; (3) respiratory distress (tachypnea, dyspnea, retraction may be signs of serious

TABLE 1–1.

Selected Syndromes and Diseases Associated With Cardiovascular Malformations

Syndrome or Disease	Common CV Malformations
Apert syndrome	VSD, TOF
Bronchopulmonary dysplasia	Cor pulmonale
Cockayne syndrome	Accelerated atherosclerosis
Crouzon disease (craniofacial dysotosis)	PDA, COA
Ehlers-Danlos syndrome	Aneurysm of aorta and carotids
Ellis–van Creveld syndrome (chondroectodermal dysplasia)	Single atrium
Friedreich ataxia	Cardiomyopathy, conduction defects
Glycogen storage disease type II (Pompe disease)	Cardiomyopathy
Goldenhar syndrome	TOF, VSD
Holt-Oram syndrome (cardiac limb)	ASD, VSD
Homocystinuria	Aortic and PA dilatation, intravascular thrombosis
Hypertrophic obstructive cardiomyopathy (HOCM)	Hypertrophic obstructive subaortic stenosis
Incontinentia pigmenti	PDA
Kartagener syndrome	Dextrocardia
Leopard syndrome (multiple lentigenes)	PS, long PR interval, cardiomyopathy

(Continued.)

TABLE 1–1 (cont.).

Syndrome or Disease	Common CV Malformations
Long QT syndrome (Jervell and Lange-Nielsen syndrome, Romano-Ward syndrome)	Long QT interval, ventricular tachyarrhythmias
Marfan syndrome	Aortic aneurysm, AR and/or MR
Mitral valve prolapse syndrome (primary)	MR, dysrrhythmias
Mucopolysaccharidosis (Hurler, Hunter, Morquio, Scheie syndromes)	AR/MR, coronary artery disease
Muscular dystrophy (Duchenne type)	Cardiomyopathy
Neurofibromatosis (von Recklinghausen disease)	PS, COA, pheochromocytoma
Noonan syndrome	PS (dystrophic pulmonary valve)
Osler-Weber-Rendu syndrome	AV fistulas (lungs and liver)
Osteogenesis imperfecta	AR
Pierre Robin syndrome	VSD, PDA, ASD, COA, or TOF
Progeria	Accelerated atherosclerosis
Pseudoxanthoma elasticum	Peripheral and coronary arterial disease
Rubinstein-Taybi syndrome	PDA, others
Sickle cell anemia	Cardiomyopathy, MR
Tuberous sclerosis	Rhabdomyoma
William syndrome	Supravalvar AS, peripheral PS

TABLE 1–2.

CHD in Selected Chromosomal Aberrations

Condition	Incidence of CHD (%)	Common Defects, in Decreasing Order of Frequency
5p– (cri du chat syndrome)	25	VSD, PDA, ASD
Trisomy 13	90	VSD, PDA, dextrocardia
Trisomy 18	99	VSD, PDA, PS
Trisomy 21 (Down syndrome)	50	ECD, VSD
Turner syndrome (XO)	35	COA, AS, ASD
Klinefelter variant (XXXXY)	15	PDA, ASD

CHD); (4) pallor (vasoconstriction from CHF, circulatory shock, or severe anemia; (5) sweat on forehead (in CHF).

2. Check for known syndromes or chromosomal abnormalities: (see Tables 1–1 and 1–2).
3. Cyanosis and clubbing. Cyanosis usually signals serious CHD. Long-standing arterial desaturation (usually more than 6 months), even of subclinical degree, results in clubbing of the fingernails and toenails.

B. Palpation:

1. Precordium:
   a. Hyperactive precordium is a characteristic of heart disease with increased volume overload (such as L–R shunt lesions, and severe valvular regurgitation).
   b. Thrill is often of real diagnostic value. Suggestive lesions according to the location of thrill are: (a) ULSB—PS, PA stenosis, and rarely PDA; (b) URSB—AS; (c) LLSB—VSD; (d) suprasternal notch—AS, occasionally PS, PDA, or COA; (e) carotid arteries—AS, COA.
2. Peripheral pulses:
   a. Note pulse rate, irregularities (arrhythmias), and volume (bounding, full, or thready).
   b. Strong arm pulses and weak leg pulses suggest COA.
   c. Right brachial artery pulse stronger than the left brachial pulse may be associated with COA or supravalvular AS.
   d. Bounding pulses are found in aortic runoff lesions (PDA, AR, large systemic AV fistula, rarely persistent truncus arteriosus).
   e. Weak, thready pulses are found in CHF or circulatory shock.
   f. Pulsus paradoxus may be seen in patients with cardiac tamponade, constrictive pericarditis and in those on a respirator with high pressure settings.

C. Blood Pressure:

Correct size of BP cuff: Cuffs that are too narrow will overestimate the true BP, and cuffs too wide will underestimate the true BP. The width of the inflatable part of the cuff (bladder) should be 125% to 155% of the diameter (or 40% to 50% of the circumference) of the limb (either arm or leg) on which BP is to be determined (Fig 1–1), as recommended by the AHA. Cuff selection based solely on the length of the arm (three fourths of the length of the upper arm as recommended by the NIH Task Force, 1987) is scientifically unsound. The cuff should be long enough to completely or nearly completely encircle the limb.

For the auscultatory method, phase I of the Korotkoff sounds is taken as systolic pressure. The points of muffling (Phase IV) are taken as diastolic pressure

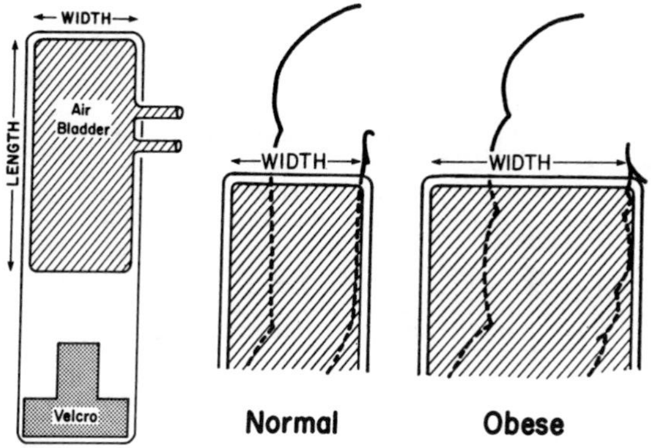

FIG 1–1.
Diagram showing a method of selecting an apppropriate-sized blood pressure cuff. (From Park MK: *Pediatric Cardiology for Practitioners,* ed 2. Chicago, Year Book Medical Publishers, 1988.)

TABLE 1–3.

Suggested Normal BP Values (mm Hg)*

Age (yr)		Mean	90th%	95th%
6–7		104/55	114/73	117/78
8–9		106/58	118/76	120/82
10–11		108/60	120/77	124/82
12–13		112/62	124/78	128/83
14–15	Boys	116/66	132/80	138/86
	Girls	112/68	126/80	130/83
16–18	Boys	121/70	136/82	140/86
	Girls	110/68	125/81	127/84

**From Park MK, Guntheroth WG:* Am J Noninvasive Cardiol *1989; 3:297–309. Used by permission.*

in children 12 years and younger and of disappearance (Phase V) in children 13 years and older, but when these are more than 6 mm Hg apart, both values should be noted (e.g., 110/75/50 mm Hg). Although there is no single reliable set of normative BP values, a working guide of normal BP values is needed until more reliable data become available (Table 1–3).

Accuracy of indirect BP measurement by an oscillometric method (Dinamap) has been demonstrated.

TABLE 1–4.

Normative Blood Pressure Levels* by Dinamap Monitor (mm Hg)

Age	Mean	90th%	95th%
1–3 days	65/41 (50)	75/49 (59)	78/52 (62)
1 mo–2 yr	95/58 (72)	106/68 (83)	110/71 (86)
2–5 yr	101/57 (74)	112/66 (82)	115/68 (85)

**Mean value in parenthesis.*

Cuff width 40% to 50% of the circumference (or 125% to 155% of the diameter) of the arm is also appropriate for the Dinamap method. Normal BP levels by the Dinamap method are presented in Table 1–4 for newborns and children to 5 years of age.

D. Auscultation:

Attention should be given systematically to (a) heart rate and regularity; (b) intensity and quality of heart sounds, especially the second heart sound; (c) systolic and diastolic sounds (ejection click, midsystolic click, opening snap); (d) heart murmurs.

1. Heart sounds:
   a. First heart sound (S1) is associated with closure of the mitral and tricuspid valves, and is best heard at the apex or LLSB. Splitting of the S1 may be found in normal children but is infrequent. Wide splitting of S1 may be found in RBBB or Ebstein anomaly.
   b. Second heart sound (S2) is evaluated in the ULSB (or pulmonary area) in terms of (a) degree of splitting and (b) relative intensity of

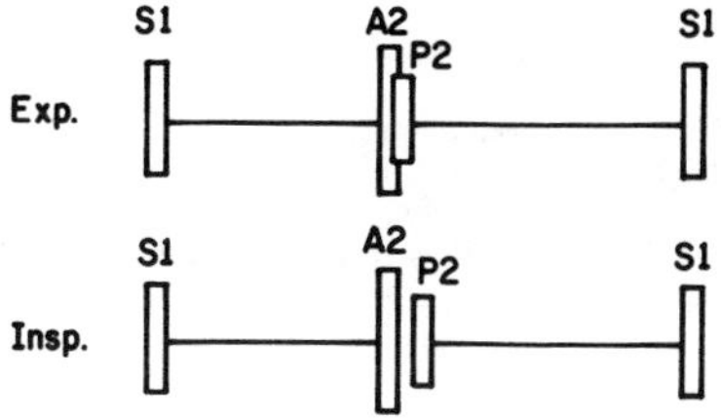

FIG 1–2.
Diagram showing relative intensity of A2 and P2 and the respiratory variation in the degree of splitting of the S2 at the ULSB (pulmonary area). (From Park MK: *Pediatric Cardiology for Practitioners,* ed 2. Chicago, Year Book Medical Publishers, 1988.)

P2 (in relation to the intensity of A2). Although best heard with a diaphragm, both components are readily audible with the bell as well.

(1) The degree of splitting of the S2 normally varies with respiration, increasing with inspiration and decreasing or becoming single with expiration (Fig 1–2).

(2) Abnormal S2 may be in the form of (a) wide splitting, (b) narrow splitting, (c) single S2, (d) abnormal intensity of P2, or

TABLE 1–5.

Summary of Abnormal S2

Abnormal splitting
1. Widely split and fixed S2
    a. Volume overload (ASD, PAPVR)
    b. Pressure overload (PS)
    c. Electrical delay (RBBB)
    d. Early aortic closure (MR)
    e. Occasional normal child
2. Narrowly split S2
    a. Pulmonary hypertension
    b. AS
    c. Occasional normal child
3. Single S2
    a. Pulmonary hypertension
    b. One semilunar valve (pulmonary atresia, aortic atresia, persistent truncus arteriosus)
    c. P2 not audible (TGA, TOF, severe PS)
    d. Severe AS
    e. Occasional normal child
4. Paradoxically split S2
    a. Severe AS
    b. LBBB, WPW syndrome (type B)

Abnormal intensity of P2
1. Increased P2 (pulmonary hypertension)
2. Decreased P2 (severe PS, TOF, tricuspid stenosis)

rarely, (e) paradoxical splitting of S2 (Table 1–5).

c. Third heart sound (S3) is best heard at the apex or LLSB (Fig 1–3). It is commonly heard in normal children, young adults, and in conditions with dilated ventricles and decreased compliance (large shunt VSD, CHF).
d. Fourth heart sound (S4) at the apex is always pathologic (see Fig 1–3) and is seen in conditions with decreased ventricular compliance or CHF.
e. Gallop rhythm generally implies a pathologic condition, and results from the combination

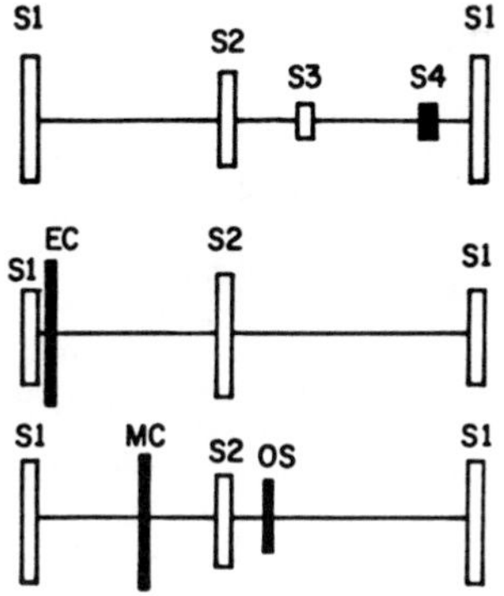

FIG 1–3.
Diagram showing the relative position of the heart sounds, ejection click *(EC)*, midsystolic click *(MC)*, and diastolic opening snap *(OS)*. Filled bars show abnormal sounds. (From Park MK: *Pediatric Cardiology for Practitioners*, ed 2. Chicago, Year Book Medical Publishers, 1988.)

of a loud S3 or S4 and tachycardia. It is commonly present in CHF.

2. Systolic and diastolic sounds:
   a. Ejection click (or ejection sound), which sounds like splitting of S1, is most audible at the base (see Fig 1–3). The ejection click is associated with the following:
      (1) PS (at 2–3 LICS) or AS (at 2 RICS or apex).
      (2) Dilated great arteries (systemic or pulmonary hypertension, idiopathic dilatation of PA, TOF [in which the aorta is dilated], and persistent truncus arteriosus).
   b. Midsystolic click with or without late systolic murmur is heard at the apex in mitral valve prolapse (see Fig 1–3).
   c. Diastolic opening snap is audible at the apex or LLSB in MS (see Fig 1–3).
3. Heart murmur:
   Each heart murmur must be analyzed in terms of intensity (grades 1 to 6), timing (systolic or diastolic), location, transmission, and quality (e.g., musical, vibratory, blowing).
      (1) Intensity of the murmur is customarily graded from 1 to 6:
      Grade 1: barely audible.
      Grade 2: soft but easily audible.
      Grade 3: moderately loud but not accompanied by a thrill.
      Grade 4: louder and associated with a thrill.
      Grade 5: audible with the stethoscope barely on the chest.
      Grade 6: audible with the stethoscope off the chest.
      (2) Classification of heart murmurs:
      Based on the timing of the heart murmur in relation to the S1 and S2, the heart murmur is classified into three types: systolic, diastolic, and continuous murmur.

a. Systolic murmur:

(1) Types of systolic murmur: A systolic murmur occurs between S1 and S2 and is classified as one of two types—ejection or regurgitant—depending on the timing of the onset of the heart murmur in relation to the S1.

(a) Ejection murmur (stenotic, diamond-shaped, crescendo-decrescendo): There is an interval between the S1 and the onset of the murmur and is crescendo–decrescendo. The murmur may be short or long (Fig 1–4,A). These murmurs are caused by flow of blood through stenotic or deformed semilunar valves or increased flow through normal semilunar valves and are therefore found at the base or over the midprecordium.

(b) Regurgitant systolic murmur: These

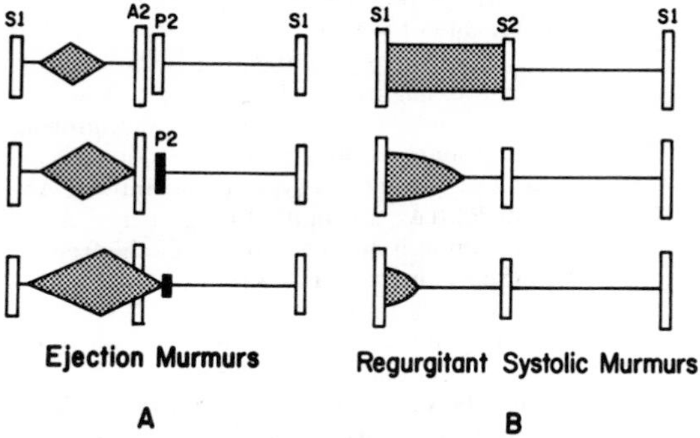

FIG 1–4.
Diagram of ejection and regurgitant systolic murmurs. (From Park MK: *Pediatric Cardiology for Practitioners,* ed 2. Chicago, Year Book Medical Publishers, 1988.)

murmurs begin with the S1 (no gap between the S1 and the murmur) and usually last throughout systole (pansystolic or holosystolic), but may be decrescendo, ending in middle or early systole (Fig 1–4,B). These murmurs are associated with only three conditions: VSD, MR, TR.

(2) Location of systolic murmurs:
In addition to the type of murmur (ejection or regurgitant), the location of the maximal intensity of the murmur is of great importance in making a clinical diagnosis of the origin of heart murmur. This important topic is discussed in detail in Tables 1–6 through 1–9 and Fig 1–5.

(3) Transmission of systolic murmurs:
A systolic ejection murmur at the base that transmits well to the neck is more likely to be aortic; one that transmits well to the back is more likely to be of pulmonary valve or pulmonary artery origin.

(4) Quality of systolic murmurs:
The quality of a murmur may be helpful in the diagnosis of heart disease. Systolic murmurs of MR or VSD have a uniform, high-pitched quality often described as blowing. Ejection systolic murmurs of AS or PS have a rough, grating quality. A common innocent murmur in children (Still's murmur) has a characteristic vibratory or humming quality.

b. Differential diagnosis of systolic murmurs at various locations:
Figure 1–5 illustrates systolic murmurs that are audible at various locations. Tables 1–6 through 1–9 summarize other important clinical findings (physical examination, chest x-ray films, and ECG) that may aid in the correct diagnosis of heart conditions according to the

TABLE 1–6.

Differential Diagnosis of Systolic Murmurs at the ULSB (Pulmonary Area)

Condition	Important Physical Findings	Chest X-ray Findings	ECG Findings
Pulmonary valve stenosis (PS)	SEM, grade 2–5/6, *Thrill (±) S2 may be split widely when mild *Ejection click (±) at 2LICS Transmit to back	*Prominent MPA (poststenotic dilatation) Normal PVM	Normal if mild, RAD *RVH RAH if severe
Atrial septal defect (ASD)	SEM, grade 2–3/6 *Widely split and fixed S2	*Increased PVM *RAE and RVE	RAD RVH *RBBB (rsR′)
Pulmonary flow murmur of newborn	SEM, grade 1–2/6 No thrill *Good transmission to back and axillae	Normal	Normal
Pulmonary flow murmur of older children	SEM, grade 2–3/6 No thrill Poor transmission	Normal Occasional pectus excavatum or straight back	Normal
Pulmonary artery stenosis	SEM, grade 2–3/6 Occasional continuous murmur P2 may be loud *Transmits well to back and both lung fields	Prominent hilar vessels (±)	RVH or normal

(Continued.)

TABLE 1–6 (cont.).

Condition	Important Physical Findings	Chest X-ray Findings	ECG Findings
Aortic stenosis (AS)	SEM, grade 2–5/6 *Also audible in 2RICS *Thrill (±) at 2RICS and SSN *Ejection click at apex, 3LICS, or 2RICS (±) Paradox split S2 if severe	Dilated aorta	Normal or LVH
Tetralogy of Fallot (TOF)	*Long SEM, grade 2–4/6 Louder at MLSB Thrill (±) Loud, single S2 (=A2) Cyanosis, clubbing	*Decreased PVM *Normal heart size Boot-shaped heart Right aortic arch (25%)	RAD *RVH or CVH RAH (±)
Coarctation of aorta (COA)	SEM, grade 1–3/6 *Loudest at left interscapular area (back) *Weak or absent femorals Hypertension in arms Frequently associated with AS, bicuspid aortic valve, or MR	*Classic "3" sign on plain film or "E" sign on barium esophagogram Rib notching (±)	LVH in children RBBB (or RVH) in newborns

Patent ductus arteriosus (PDA)	*Continuous murmur, at left infraclavicular area Occasional crescendic systolic only Grade 2–4/6 Thrill (±) Bounding pulses	*Increased PVM *LAE, LVE	Normal, LVH, or CVH
Total anomalous pulmonary venous return (TAPVR)	SEM, grade 2–3/6 Widely split and fixed S2 (±) *Quadruple or quintuple rhythm Diastolic rumble at LLSB *Mild cyanosis and clubbing (±)	*Increased PVM RAE and RVE Prominent MPA "Snowman" sign	RAD RAH *RVH
Partial anomalous pulmonary venous return (PAPVR)	Physical findings similar to those of ASD *S2 may not be fixed unless associated with ASD	*Increased PVM *RAE and RVE "Scimitar" sign (±)	Same as in ASD

**Finding is particularly characteristic of the condition.*

AS = aortic stenosis; CVH = combined ventricular hypertrophy; 2LICS = second left intercostal space; LLSB = lower left sternal border, MLSB = mid-left sternal border; LVE = left ventricular enlargement; LVH = left ventricular hypertrophy; MPA = main pulmonary artery; MR = mitral regurgitation; PVM = pulmonary vascular markings; RAD = right axis deviation; RAE = right atrial enlargement; RAH = right atrial hypertrophy; RBBB = right bundle branch block; RVE = right ventricular enlargement; RVH = right ventricular hypertrophy; SEM = systolic ejection murmur, SSN = suprasternal notch.

TABLE 1–7.

Differential Diagnosis of Systolic Murmurs at the URSB (Aortic Area)

Condition	Important Physical Findings	Chest X-ray Findings	ECG Findings
Aortic valve stenosis	SEM, grade 2–5/6, at 2RICS, may be loudest at 3LICS *Thrill (±), URSB, SSN, and carotid arteries *Ejection click *Transmits well to neck S2 may be single	Mild LVE (±) Prominent ascending aorta or aortic knob	Normal or LVH with or without "strain"
Subaortic stenosis	SEM, grade 2–4/6 *AR murmur usually present No ejection click	Usually normal	Normal or LVH

Supravalvular aortic stenosis	SEM, grade 2–3/6 Thrill (±) No ejection click *Pulse and BP may be greater in R than L arm *Peculiar facies, and mental retardation (±) Murmur may transmit well to back (PA stenosis)	Unremarkable	Normal, LVH or CVH

**Finding is particularly characteristic of the condition.*

AR = aortic regurgitation; CVH = combined ventricular hypertrophy; 3LICS = third left intercostal space; LVE = left ventricular enlargement; LVH = left ventricular hypertrophy; PA = pulmonary artery; 2RICS = second right intercostal space; SEM = systolic ejection murmur; SSN = suprasternal notch; URSB = upper right sternal border.

TABLE 1–8.

Differential Diagnosis of Systolic Murmurs at the LLSB

Condition	Important Physical Findings	Chest X-ray Findings	ECG Findings
Ventricular septal defect (VSD)	*Regurgitant systolic, grade 2–5/6 May not be holosystolic Well-localized at LLSB *Thrill often present P2 may be loud	*Increased PVM *LAE and LVE (cardiomegaly)	Normal LVH or CVH
Endocardial cushion defect, complete (ECD)	Similar to findings of VSD *Diastolic rumble at LLSB *Gallop rhythm common in infants (CHF)	Similar to large VSD	*Superior QRS axis, LVH or CVH
Vibratory innocent murmur (Still's)	SEM, grade 2–3/6 *Musical or vibratory with midsystolic accentuation *Maximum between LLSB and apex	Normal	Normal

Hypertrophic obstructive cardiomyopathy (HOCM or IHSS)	SEM, grade 2–4/6 Medium-pitched Maximum LLSB or apex Thrill (±) *Sharp upstroke of brachial pulses May have MR murmur	Normal or globular LVE	LVH Abnormally deep Q waves in V5 and V6
Tricuspid regurgitation (TR)	*Regurgitant systolic, grade 2–3/6 *Triple or quadruple rhythm (in Ebstein anomaly) Mild cyanosis (±) Hepatomegaly with pulsatile liver and neck vein distention when severe	Normal PVM RAE if severe	RBBB, RAH, and first-degree AV block in Ebstein anomaly
Tetralogy of Fallot (TOF)	(See Table 2–5) Murmurs can be louder at ULSB		

Finding is characteristic of the condition.
CHF = congestive heart failure; CVH = combined ventricular hypertrophy; ECD = endocardial cushion defect; IHSS = idiopathic hypertrophic subaortic stenosis; LAE = left atrial enlargement; LLSB = lower left sternal border; LVE = left ventricular enlargement; LVH = left ventricular hypertrophy; MR = mitral regurgitation; PVM = pulmonary vascular markings; RAE = right atrial enlargement; RAH = right atrial hypertrophy; RBBB = right bundle branch block; ULSB = upper left sternal border; VSD = ventricular septal defect.

TABLE 1–9.

Differential Diagnosis of Systolic Murmurs at the Apex

Condition	Important Physical Findings	Chest X-ray Findings	ECG Findings
Mitral regurgitation (MR)	*Regurgitant systolic, may not be holosystolic, grade 2–3/6 Transmits to left axilla (less obvious in children) May be loudest in the mid-precordium	LAE and LVE	LAH or LVH
Mitral valve prolapse (MVP)	*Midsystolic click with or without late systolic murmur *High incidence (85%) of thoracic skeletal anomalies (e.g., pectus excavatum, straight back)	Normal	Inverted T in aVF

Aortic valve stenosis (AS)	Murmur and ejection click may be best heard at apex rather than at 2RICS	(See Table 1–7)
Hypertrophic obstructive cardiomyopathy (HOCM or IHSS)	Murmur of IHSS may be maximal at apex (may represent MR) (See Table 1–8)	
Vibratory innocent murmur	This innocent murmur may be loudest at apex (See Table 1–8)	

**Finding is characteristic of the condition.*
IHSS = idiopathic hypertrophic subaortic stenosis; LAE = left atrial enlargement; LAH = left atrial hypertrophy; LVE = left ventricular enlargement; LVH = left ventricular hypertrophy; MR = mitral regurgitation; 2RICS = second right intercostal space.

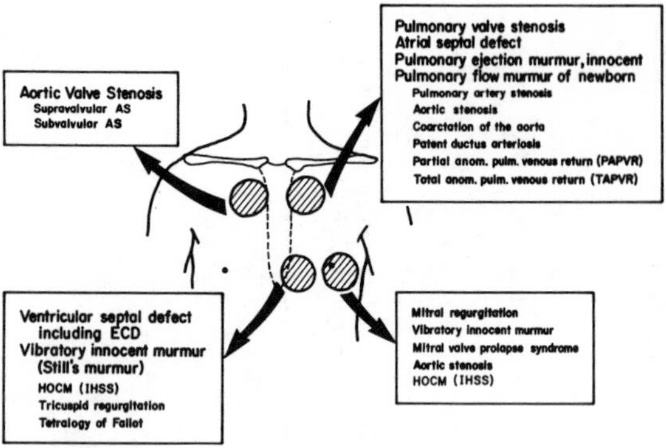

FIG 1–5.
Diagram showing systolic murmurs audible at various locations. Less common conditions are shown in smaller type (see Tables 1–6 through 1–9). (From Park MK: *Pediatric Cardiology for Practitioners,* ed 2. Chicago, Year Book Medical Publishers, 1988.)

location of systolic murmurs.

c. Diastolic murmurs:
Diastolic murmurs occur between S2 and S1, and are classified into three types:
(1) Early diastolic (protodiastolic) decrescendo murmurs are caused by incompetence of the aortic or pulmonary valve (Fig 1–6). AR murmurs are high pitched, are best heard with the diaphragm of the stethoscope at the 3LICS, and radiate to the apex. PR murmurs are usually medium pitched, but may be high pitched if pulmonary hypertension is present, are best heard at the 2LICS, and radiate along the left sternal border.

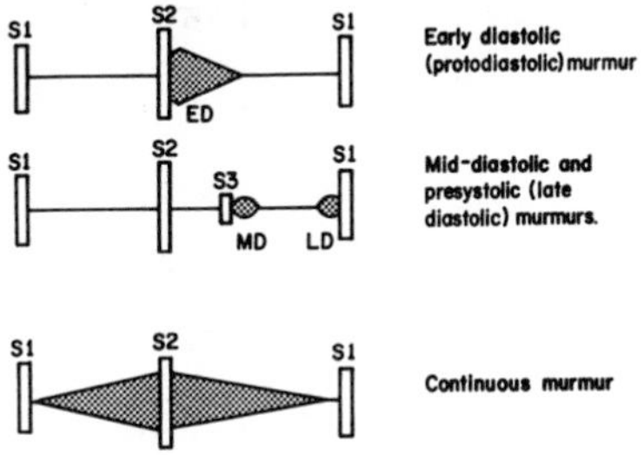

FIG 1–6.
Diagram of diastolic murmurs and the continuous murmur. (From Park MK: *Pediatric Cardiology for Practitioners,* ed 2. Chicago, Year Book Medical Publishers, 1988.)

(2) Mid-diastolic murmurs are always low pitched, start with a loud S3 (see Fig 1–6), and are best heard with the bell of the stethoscope. These murmurs are caused by anatomic stenosis or relative stenosis of the mitral or tricuspid valves. MS murmurs are best heard at the apex (apical rumble), and TS murmurs are heard along the LLSB.

(3) Presystolic (or late diastolic) murmurs are low pitched and occur late in diastole or just before the onset of systole (see Fig 1–6) and are found with anatomic stenosis of the mitral or tricuspid valve.

d. Continuous murmur:
Continuous murmurs begin in systole and continue without interruption through the S2 into all or part of diastole (see Fig 1–6). Continuous murmurs can be caused by:
(1) Aortopulmonary or arteriovenous connec-

TABLE 1–10.

Common Innocent Heart Murmurs

Type (Timing)	Description of Murmur	Age Group
Classic vibratory murmur (Still's murmur) (Systolic)	Maximal at MLSB or between LLSB and apex Grade 2–3/6 Low-frequency vibratory, "twanging string," groaning, squeaking, or musical	3–6 yr Occasionally in infancy
Pulmonary ejection murmur (Systolic)	Maximal at ULSB Early to midsystolic Grade 1–3/6 in intensity Blowing in quality	8–14 yr

Pulmonary flow murmur of newborn (Systolic)	Maximal at ULSB Transmits well to left and right chest, axillae, and back Grade 1–2/6 in intensity	Premature and full-term newborns Usually disappears by 3–6 mo of age
Venous hum (continuous)	Maximal at right (or left supraclavicular and infraclavicular areas) Grade 1–3/6 in intensity Inaudible in supine position Intensity changes with rotation of head and compression of jugular vein	3–6 yr
Carotid bruit (Systolic)	Right supraclavicular area and over carotids Grade 2–3/6 in intensity Occasional thrill over carotid	Any age

tion (PDA, AV fistula, or after S–P shunt surgery, or rarely, persistent truncus arteriosus).

(2) Disturbances of flow patterns in veins (venous hum).

(3) Disturbance of flow pattern in arteries (COA, peripheral PA stenosis).

The combination of a systolic and a diastolic murmur, such as from AS and AR or PS and PR, is referred to as a to-and-fro murmur to distinguish it from a machinery-like continuous murmur.

e. Innocent heart murmurs:
More than 80% of children will have innocent murmurs of one type or the other sometime during childhood, most commonly beginning at about 3 or 4 years of age. All innocent heart murmurs are accentuated or brought out in high-output states, most importantly with fever, and are associated with normal ECG and x-ray findings. Clinical characteristics of these murmurs are summarized in Table 1–10.

When one or more of the following are present, the murmur is more likely pathologic and will require cardiac consultation: (1) symptoms, (2) cyanosis, (3) abnormal chest x-ray film (heart size, silhouette and pulmonary vascularity), (4) abnormal ECG, (5) systolic murmur that is loud (grade 3/6 or with thrill) and long, (6) diastolic murmur, (7) abnormal heart sounds, and (8) abnormally strong or weak pulses.

III. ELECTROCARDIOGRAPHY

Normal Pediatric Electrocardiograms

Electrocardiograms of normal infants and children are different from those of normal adults; they show RV dominance most marked in the newborn. RV dominance of infants is expressed in the ECG by:

1. Right-axis deviation
2. Large rightward forces (tall R waves in aVR and the right precordial leads [RPLs such as V4R, V1, and V2], and deep S waves in lead I and the left precordial leads [LPLs such as V5 and V6])

A. Routine Interpretation:

The following sequence is one of many approaches that can be used in routine interpretation of an ECG:

a. Rhythm (sinus or nonsinus) by considering the P axis.
b. Heart rate (atrial and ventricular rates, if different).
c. QRS axis, T axis, and QRS-T angle.
d. PR, QRS, and QT intervals.
e. P wave amplitude and duration.
f. QRS amplitude and R/S ratio; also note abnormal Q waves.
g. ST segment and T wave abnormalities.

1. Rhythm

Sinus rhythm is the normal rhythm at any age and is characterized by:

a. P wave preceding each QRS complex with a regular PR interval.
b. P axis between 0 and +90 degrees (upright P in I and aVF).

2. Heart rate

At the usual paper speed of 25/mm sec, 1 mm = 0.04 sec, and 5 mm = 0.20 sec.

a. Measure the RR interval (in seconds), then divide 60 by the RR interval.
b. A quick estimation of heart rate is possible by inspecting the RR interval in millimeters and using the following relationship; 5 mm—300/sec, 10 mm—150/sec, 15 mm—100/sec, 20 mm—75/sec, 25 mm—60/sec (Fig 1–7).
c. Use a convenient ECG ruler.

Normal resting heart rates per minute according to age

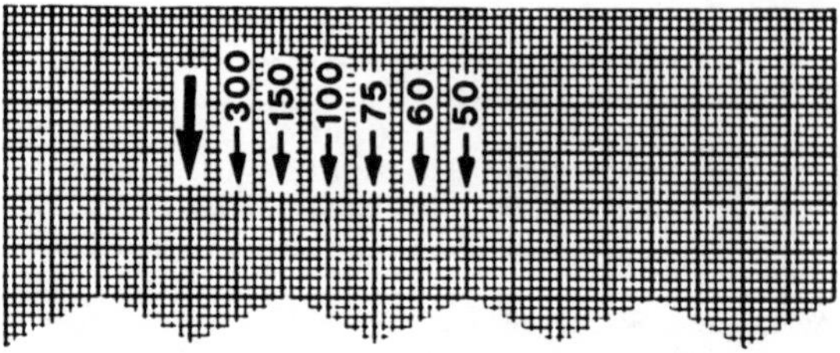

FIG 1–7.
Quick method for estimating heart rate.

are as follows: Newborn—110–150; 2 years old—85–125; 4 years old—75–115; and >6 years old—60–100.

Tachycardia is present when the heart rate is faster than the upper range of normal, and bradycardia is present when the heart rate is slower than the lower range of normal for that age.

3. QRS axis, T axis, and QRS-T angle:

a. QRS axis: The most convenient way of deter-

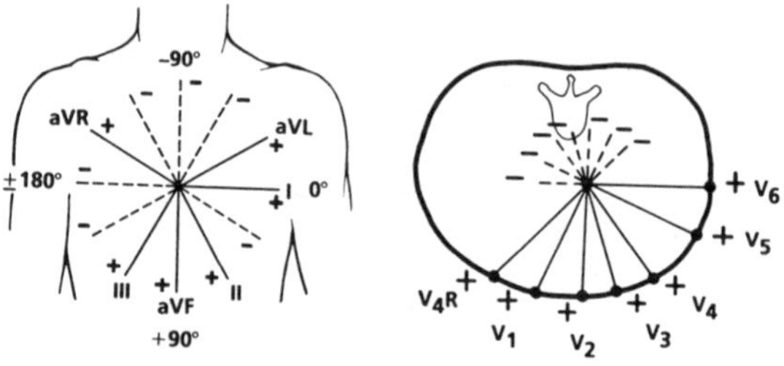

FIG 1–8.
Hexaxial reference system *(left)* and horizontal reference system *(right)*. (From Park MK: Guntheroth WG: *How to Read Pediatric ECGs*, ed 2. Chicago, Year Book Medical Publishers, 1987.)

mining the QRS axis is by the use of the **hexaxial reference system** (Fig 1–8,A), which gives information about the left-right and superior-inferior relationship. The R wave in lead I represents the leftward force, and the S wave in lead I the rightward force. The R wave in aVF is the inferior force, and the S wave the superior force.

Successive Approximation Method:

Step 1: Locate a quadrant, using leads I and aVF (Fig 1–9).

Step 2: Find a lead with equiphasic QRS complex (in which the height of the R wave and the depth of the S wave are equal). The QRS axis is perpendicular to the lead with equiphasic QRS complex in the predetermined quadrant.

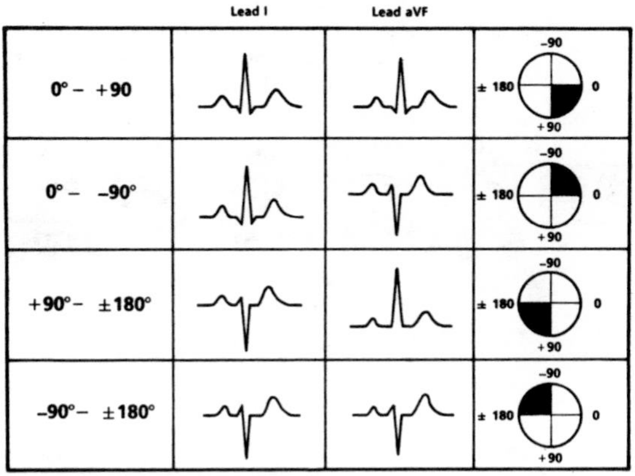

FIG 1–9.
Locating quadrants of mean QRS axis from leads I and aVF. (From Park MK, Guntheroth WG: *How to Read Pediatric ECGs,* ed 2. Chicago, Year Book Medical Publishers, 1987.)

EXAMPLE: Determine the QRS axis in Fig 1–10:

Step 1: The axis is in the left lower quadrant (0 to +90 degrees), because the R waves are upright in both leads I and aVF.

Step 2: The QRS complex is equiphasic in aVL. Therefore the QRS axis is +60 degrees, which is perpendicular to aVL.

(1) Normal ranges of QRS axis vary with age (Table 1–11).

(2) Abnormal QRS axis:

(a) LAD occurs with LVH, LBBB, and left anterior hemiblock (or "superior" QRS axis).

(b) RAD occurs with RVH and RBBB.

(c) "Superior QRS" axis is present when the S wave is greater than the R wave in aVF. It may occur with left anterior hemiblock (in the range of −30 to −90 degrees) or with RBBB.

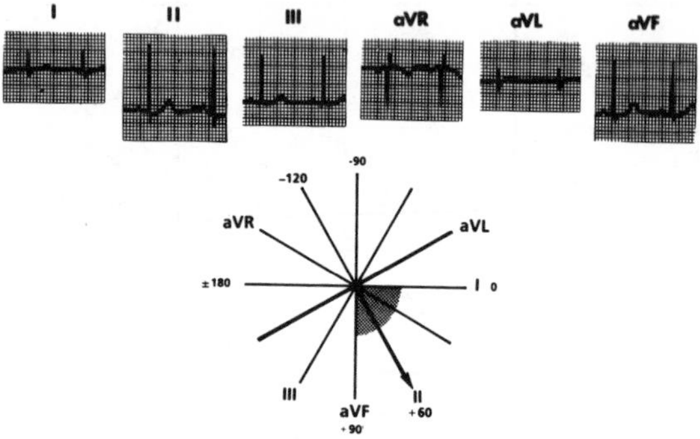

FIG 1–10.
Example of determination of QRS axis (see text).

TABLE 1–11.

Mean and Range of Normal QRS Axes

1 wk–1 mo	+110 degrees (+30–+180)
1–3 mo	+70 degrees (+10–+125)
3 mo–3 yr	+60 degrees (+10–+110)
>3 yr	+60 degrees (+20–+120)
Adults	+50 degrees (−30–+105)

Horizontal Reference System:
Whereas the hexaxial reference system gives information about the left-right and superior-inferior relationships, the horizontal reference system gives information about the anteroposterior and left-right relationship. The horizontal reference system utilizes precordial leads (see Fig 1–8,B).

b. T axis: The T axis can be determined by the same methods used to determine the QRS axis.
   (1) Normal T axis: 0 degrees to +90 degrees.
   (2) Abnormal T axis (outside 0 degrees to +90 degrees quadrant) suggests conditions with myocardial dysfunction (myocarditis, myocardial ischemia), ventricular hypertrophy with "strain," or RBBB.
c. The QRS-T angle is formed by the QRS axis and the T axis.
   (1) Normal QRS-T angle is less than 60 degrees.
   (2) Abnormal QRS-T angle (more than 90 degrees) is seen in severe ventricular hypertrophy with "strain," ventricular conduction disturbances, and metabolic or ischemic myocardial dysfunction.

4. Intervals:
   a. PR interval: Normal PR interval varies with age and heart rate (Table 1–12).
      (1) A prolonged PR interval (first-degree AV

TABLE 1–12.

PR Interval With Rate and Age (and Upper Limits of Normal)*

Rate	0–1 mo	1–6 mo	6 mo–1 yr	1–3 yr	3–8 yr	8–12 yr	12–16 yr	Adult
<60						0.16 (0.18)	0.16 (0.19)	0.17 (0.21)
60–80					0.15 (0.17)	0.15 (0.17)	0.15 (0.18)	0.16 (0.21)
80–100	0.10 (0.12)				0.14 (0.16)	0.15 (0.16)	0.15 (0.17)	0.15 (0.20)
100–120	0.10 (0.12)			(0.15)	0.13 (0.16)	0.14 (0.15)	0.15 (0.16)	0.15 (0.19)
120–140	0.10 (0.11)	0.11 (0.14)	0.11 (0.14)	0.12 (0.14)	0.13 (0.15)	0.14 (0.15)		0.15 (0.18)
140–160	0.09 (0.11)	0.10 (0.13)	0.11 (0.13)	0.11 (0.14)	0.12 (0.14)			(0.17)
160–180	0.10 (0.11)	0.10 (0.12)	0.10 (0.12)	0.10 (0.12)				
>180	0.09	0.09 (0.11)	0.10 (0.11)					

**From Park MK, Guntheroth WG:* How to Read Pediatric ECGs, *ed 2. Chicago, Year Book Medical Publishers, 1987.*

block) may be seen in myocarditis (viral or rheumatic), certain CHD (ECD, ASD, Ebstein anomaly), digitalis toxicity, hyperkalemia, other myocardial dysfunction, and also in an otherwise normal heart.

(2) A short PR interval is present in preexcitation (WPW syndrome, Lown-Ganong-Levine syndrome) and glycogen storage disease.

b. QRS Duration: Normal QRS duration varies with age (Table 1–13). A long QRS duration is characteristic of ventricular conduction disturbances (BBBs, preexcitation, intraventricular block, ventricular arrhythmias) and is rarely seen in ventricular hypertrophy.

c. QT Interval: The QT interval normally varies primarily with heart rate (Table 1–14). The heart rate corrected QT interval (QTc) can be calculated by the use of Bazett's formula:

$$QTc = QT\ \text{measured}/\sqrt{\text{RR interval}}$$

(1) Normal QTc does not exceed 0.425 second, except in infants. QTc up to 0.49 sec may be normal for the first 6 months of age.

(2) Long QT intervals may be seen in conditions such as hypocalcemia, myocarditis, diffuse myocardial diseases, long QT syndrome (Jervell and Lange-Nielsen syndrome, Romano-Ward syndrome), and head injury.

(3) A short QT interval is a sign of digitalis effect or hypercalcemia.

5. P wave duration and amplitude:
Normally the P amplitude is less than 3 mm. The duration of the P waves is shorter than 0.09 sec in children, and shorter than 0.07 sec in infants.

TABLE 1–13.

QRS Duration: Average (and Upper Limits) for Age*

	0–1 mo	1–6 mo	6 mo–1 yr	1–3 yr	3–8 yr	8–12 yr	12–16 yr	Adult
Seconds	0.05 (0.07)	0.05 (0.07)	0.05 (0.07)	0.06 (0.07)	0.07 (0.08)	0.07 (0.09)	0.07 (0.10)	0.08 (0.10)

* *Modified from Guntheroth WG:* Pediatric Electrocardiography. *Philadelphia, WB Saunders Co, 1965.*

TABLE 1–14.

Cycle Length, Heart Rate, and QT Interval Average (and Upper Limits)*

Cycle Length (sec)	Heart Rate (per min)	QT Interval (sec)	Cycle Length (sec)	Heart Rate (per min)	QT Interval (sec)
1.50	40	0.45 (0.49)	0.85	70	0.36 (0.38)
1.40	43	0.44 (0.48)	0.80	75	0.35 (0.38)
1.30	46	0.43 (0.47)	0.75	80	0.34 (0.37)
1.25	48	0.42 (0.46)	0.70	86	0.33 (0.36)
1.20	50	0.41 (0.45)	0.65	92	0.32 (0.35)
1.15	52	0.41 (0.45)	0.60	100	0.31 (0.34)
1.10	55	0.40 (0.44)	0.55	109	0.30 (0.33)
1.05	57	0.39 (0.43)	0.50	120	0.28 (0.31)
1.00	60	0.39 (0.42)	0.45	133	0.27 (0.29)
0.95	63	0.38 (0.41)	0.40	150	0.25 (0.28)
0.90	67	0.37 (0.40)	0.35	172	0.23 (0.26)

**From Guntheroth WG:* Pediatric Electrocardiography. *Philadelphia, WB Saunders Co, 1965. Used by permission.*

(1) Tall P waves are indicative of right atrial hypertrophy (RAH).
(2) Long P wave durations are seen in left atrial hypertrophy (LAH).

6. QRS amplitude, R/S ratio, and abnormal Q waves:
   a. QRS amplitude varies with age (Table 1–15).
      (1) Large QRS amplitudes are found in ventricular hypertrophy and ventricular conduction disturbances (e.g., BBB, WPW syndrome).
      (2) Low QRS voltages are seen in pericarditis, myocarditis, and hypothyroidism, and are normal in newborns.
   b. In normal infants and small children the R/S ratio is large in the RPLs and small in the LPLs, because of tall R waves in the RPLs and deep S waves in the LPLs (Table 1–16).
      Abnormal R/S ratios are seen in ventricular hypertrophy and ventricular conduction disturbances.
   c. Normal Q waves are narrow (0.02 sec in duration) and are usually less than 5 mm in LPLs and aVF. They may be as deep as 8 mm in lead III in children younger than 3 years. Q waves are normally absent in RPLs.
      (1) Deep Q waves may be present in LPLs in ventricular hypertrophy of "volume overload" type.
      (2) Deep and wide Q waves are seen in myocardial infarction and myocardial fibrosis.
      (3) Q waves in V1 may be seen in severe RVH, ventricular inversion (L-TGA), and single ventricle and occasionally in newborns.
      (4) Absent Q waves in V6 may be seen in LBBB and ventricular inversion.
7. ST segment and T waves
   a. ST Segment: The normal ST segment is isoelectric. However, in infants and children, ele-

TABLE 1–15.

R and S Voltages According to Lead and Age: Mean (Upper Limits)*†

Voltage	Lead	0–1 mo	1–6 mo	6 mo–1 yr	1–3 yr	3–8 yr	8–12 yr	12–16 yr	Young Adults
R wave	I	4 (8)	7 (13)	8 (16)	8 (16)	7 (15)	7 (15)	6 (13)	6 (13)
	II	6 (14)	13 (24)	13 (27)	13 (23)	13 (22)	14 (24)	14 (24)	9 (25)
	III	8 (16)	9 (20)	9 (20)	9 (20)	9 (20)	9 (24)	9 (24)	6 (22)
	aVR	3 (7)	3 (6)	3 (6)	2 (6)	2 (5)	2 (4)	2 (4)	1 (4)
	aVL	2 (7)	4 (8)	5 (10)	5 (10)	3 (10)	3 (10)	3 (12)	3 (9)
	aVF	7 (14)	10 (20)	10 (16)	8 (20)	10 (19)	10 (20)	11 (21)	5 (23)
	V4R	6 (12)	5 (10)	4 (8)	4 (8)	3 (8)	3 (7)	3 (7)	
	V1	15 (25)	11 (20)	10 (20)	9 (18)	7 (18)	6 (16)	5 (16)	3 (14)
	V2	21 (30)	21 (30)	19 (28)	16 (25)	13 (28)	10 (22)	9 (19)	6 (21)
	V5	12 (30)	17 (30)	18 (30)	19 (36)	21 (36)	22 (36)	18 (33)	12 (33)
	V6	6 (21)	10 (20)	13 (20)	13 (24)	14 (24)	14 (24)	14 (22)	10 (21)
S wave	I	5 (10)	4 (9)	4 (9)	3 (8)	2 (8)	2 (8)	2 (8)	1 (6)
	V4R	4 (9)	4 (12)	5 (12)	5 (12)	5 (14)	6 (20)	6 (20)	
	V1	10 (20)	7 (18)	8 (16)	13 (27)	14 (30)	16 (26)	15 (24)	10 (23)
	V2	20 (35)	16 (30)	17 (30)	21 (34)	23 (38)	23 (38)	23 (48)	14 (36)
	V5	9 (30)	9 (26)	8 (20)	6 (16)	5 (14)	5 (17)	5 (16)	
	V6	4 (12)	2 (7)	2 (6)	2 (6)	1 (5)	1 (4)	1 (5)	1 (13)

**Modified from Park MK, Guntheroth WG*: How to Read Pediatric ECGs, ed 2. *Chicago, Year Book Medical Publishers, 1987.*

†Voltages measured in millimeters, when 1 mV = 10 mm paper.

TABLE 1–16.

R/S Ratio According to Age: Mean, Lower, and Upper Limits of Normal

	Lead	0–1 mo	1–6 mo	6 mo–1 yr	1–3 yr	3–8 yr	8–12 yr	12–16 yr	Adult
V1	LLN	0.5	0.3	0.3	0.5	0.1	0.15	0.1	0.0
	Mean	1.5	1.5	1.2	0.8	0.65	0.5	0.3	0.3
	ULN	19	S = 0	6	2	2	1	1	1
V2	LLN	0.3	0.3	0.3	0.3	0.05	0.1	0.1	0.1
	Mean	1	1.2	1	0.8	0.5	0.5	0.5	0.2
	ULN	3	4	4	1.5	1.5	1.2	1.2	2.5
V6	LLN	0.1	1.5	2	3	2.5	4	2.5	2.5
	Mean	2	4	6	20	20	20	10	9
	ULN	S = 0	S = 0	S = 0	S = 0	S = 0	S = 0	S = 0	S = 0

**From Guntheroth WG:* Pediatric Electrocardiography. *Philadelphia, WB Saunders Co, 1965. Used by permission.*
LLN = Lower limits of normal; ULN = upper limits of normal.

vation or depression of the ST segment up to 1 mm in the limb leads and up to 2 mm in the precordial leads is not necessarily abnormal.

Abnormal shift of ST segment occurs in conditions such as pericarditis, myocardial ischemia or infarction, and digitalis effect. Associated T wave changes are commonly present.

b. T Wave Amplitude: Tall, peaked T waves may be seen in hyperkalemia, LVH ("volume overload"), and cerebrovascular accident (CVA). Flat or low T waves may occur in normal newborns or in conditions such as hypothyroidism, hypokalemia, digitalis, pericarditis, myocarditis, myocardial ischemia, etc.

B. Atrial Hypertrophy:

Abnormalities in the P wave amplitude or duration are noted in atrial hypertrophy.

1. RAH—tall P waves (>3 mm).
2. LAH—wide P wave duration (>0.10 sec in children and 0.08 sec in infants).
3. Combined atrial hypertrophy (CAH)—a combination of tall and wide P waves.

C. Ventricular Hypertrophy:

Ventricular hypertrophy produces abnormalities in one or more of the following areas: QRS axis, QRS voltages, R/S ratio, T axis, and miscellaneous areas.

a. QRS axis is usually directed toward the ventricle that is hypertrophied.
b. QRS voltages increase toward the direction of the respective hypertrophied ventricle.
c. An increase in the R/S ratio in the RPLs suggests RVH, and a decrease suggests LVH. An increase in the R/S ratio in the LPLs suggests LVH, and a decrease suggests RVH (see Table 1–16).
d. Changes in the T axis are seen in severe ventricular hypertrophy with relative ischemia of the hypertrophied myocardium. In the pres-

ence of other criteria of ventricular hypertrophy, a wide QRS-T angle (90 degrees or greater) with the T axis outside the normal range indicates "strain" pattern. When the T axis remains in the normal quadrant (0 degrees to +90 degrees), a wide QRS-T angle indicates a possible "strain" pattern.

e. Miscellaneous nonspecific changes:
   RVH: (a) A q wave in V1 (either qR or qRs) is suggestive of RVH.
   (b) An upright T wave in V1 after 3 days of age is a sign of probable RVH.
   LVH: Deep Q waves (≥5 mm) or tall T waves in V5 and V6 are signs of LVH of "volume overload" type.

1. Criteria for right ventricular hypertrophy (RVH):
   a. RAD for the patient age (see Table 1–11).
   b. Increased rightward and anterior QRS voltages.
      (1) R in V1, V2, or aVR greater than ULN for patient age (see Table 1–15).
      (2) S in I and V6 greater than ULN for patient age (see Table 1–15).
   c. Abnormal R/S ratio in favor of the RV, in the absence of BBB (see Table 1–16).
      (1) R/S ratio in V1 and V2 greater than ULN for age.
      (2) R/S ratio in V6 less than 1 after 1 month of age.
   d. Upright T in V1 in patients more than 3 days of age, provided the T is upright in the LPLs (V5, V6). Upright T in V1 is not abnormal in patients 6 years or older.
   e. A q wave in V1 (qR or qRs patterns) is suggestive of RVH.
   f. In the presence of RVH, a wide QRS-T angle with T axis outside the normal range, usually in the 0 degrees to −90 degrees quadrant, indicates "strain" pattern.

2. RVH in the newborn:
   The diagnosis of RVH in the newborn is particularly difficult because of the normal dominance of the RV during that period of life. The following clues, however, are helpful in the diagnosis of RVH in newborn infants.
   a. Pure R wave (with no S wave) in V1 greater than 10 mm.
   b. R in V1 greater than 25 mm, or R in aVR greater than 8 mm.
   c. A qR pattern in V1 (also seen in 10% of healthy newborn infants).
   d. Upright T in V1 in neonates more than 3 days of age (with upright T in V6) is strongly suggestive of RVH.
   e. RAD greater than +180 degrees.
3. Criteria for left ventricular hypertrophy (LVH):
   a. LAD for the patient's age (see Table 1–11).
   b. QRS voltages in favor of the LV:
      (1) R in I, II, III, aVL, aVF, V5 or V6 greater than ULN for age (see Table 1–15).
      (2) S in V1 or V2 greater than ULN for age (see Table 1–15).
   c. Abnormal R/S ratio in favor of the LV:
      (1) R/S ratio in V1 and V2 less than LLN for patient age (see Table 1–16).
   d. Q in V5 and V6 5 mm or greater, coupled with tall symmetric T waves in the same leads (LV "volume overload").
   e. In the presence of LVH, a wide QRS-T angle with the T axis outside the normal range indicates "strain" pattern. This is manifested by flat or inverted T waves in lead I or aVF.
4. Criteria for combined ventricular hypertrophy (CVH):
   a. Positive voltage criteria for RVH and LVH (in the absence of BBB or preexcitation).
   b. Positive voltage criteria for RVH or LVH and relatively large voltages for the other ventricle.

c. Large equiphasic QRS complexes in two or more of the limb leads and in the midprecordial leads (V2 through V5), called Katz-Wachtel phenomenon.

D. Ventricular Conduction Disturbances:
Conditions that are grouped together as ventricular conduction disturbances have in common abnormal *prolongation of QRS duration* (Fig 1–11). Ventricular conduction disturbances (and their characteristic findings) include:

a. Bundle branch blocks, right and left (with the prelongation in the terminal portion of the QRS complex ["terminal slurring"]) (Fig 1–11,B).
b. Preexcitation (WPW syndrome) (with the "initial slurring" or "delta wave") (Fig 1–11,C).
c. Intraventricular block (with the prolongation throughout the QRS complex) (Fig 1–11,D).

Note that the normal QRS duration varies with age (Table 1–13). In infants, a QRS duration of 0.08 sec (not 0.10 sec as in adults) meets the requirement for BBB.

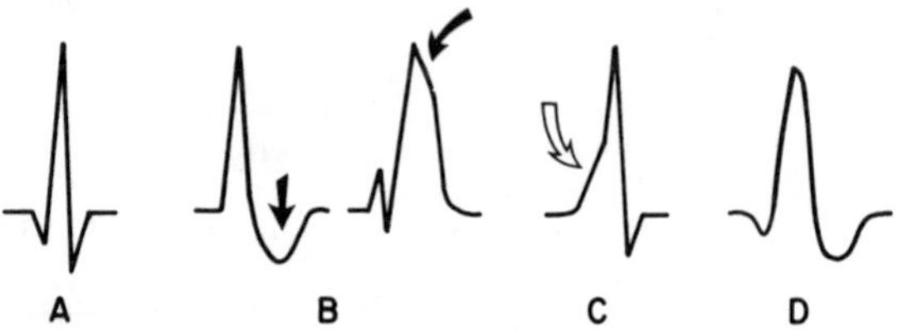

FIG 1–11.
Schematic diagram of three types of ventricular conduction disturbances. **A,** normal QRS complex. **B,** QRS complexes in RBBB with terminal slurring *(black arrows).* **C,** preexcitation with delta wave *(initial slurring, open arrow).* **D,** intraventricular block in which the prolongation of the QRS complex is throughout the duration of the QRS complex. (From Park MK: *Pediatric Cardiology for Practitioners,* ed 2. Chicago, Year Book Medical Publishers, 1988.)

1. Criteria for right bundle branch block (RBBB)
   a. RAD, at least for terminal portion of QRS complex.
   b. QRS duration longer than the ULN for patient age (see Table 1–13).
   c. Terminal slurring of the QRS complex directed to the *right* and usually, but not always, *anteriorly:*
      (1) Wide and slurred S in I, V5, and V6
      (2) Terminal, slurred R′ in aVR and the RPLs (V4R, V1 and V2).
   d. ST segment shift and T wave inversion are common in adults but not in children.
   e. It is unsafe to make a diagnosis of ventricular hypertrophy in the presence of RBBB. Because there is asynchrony of the opposing electromotive forces of each ventricle in RBBB, a greater manifest potential for both ventricles results.

   Two most common pediatric conditions that present with RBBB are ASD and conduction disturbances following open heart surgery involving right ventriculotomy. Other conditions that are often associated with RBBB include Ebstein anomaly, COA in infants younger than 6 months of age, ECD, and PAPVR, and RBBB is occasionally seen in normal children. The significance of RBBB in children is different from that in adults; in many pediatric examples of RBBB the right bundle is intact.

   Although the rsR′ pattern in V1 is unusual in adults, it is *normal* in infants and small children, provided that:
   a. QRS duration is not prolonged.
   b. Voltage of the primary or secondary R waves is not abnormally large.
2. Intraventricular block
   In this condition the prolongation is throughout the duration of the QRS complex (see Fig 1–

11,D). It is associated with metabolic disorders (hyperkalemia), myocardial ischemia (during CPR), quinidine or procainamide toxicity, and diffuse myocardial diseases (myocardial fibrosis, systemic diseases with myocardial involvement).

3. Wolff-Parkinson-White syndrome
The WPW syndrome results from an anomalous conduction pathway (bundle of Kent) between the atrium and the ventricle, bypassing the normal delay of conduction in the AV node. Patients with WPW syndrome are prone to attacks of paroxysmal supraventricular tachycardia. In the presence of this syndrome, diagnosis of ventricular hypertrophy cannot be made safely.
Criteria for WPW syndrome:
   a. Short PR interval, less than the LLN for patient age (LLN PR interval: <3 years, 0.08 sec; 3–16 years, 0.10 sec; >16 years, 0.12 sec).
   b. Delta wave (initial slurring of the QRS complex).
   c. Wide QRS duration (beyond ULN).

   There are two other forms of preexcitation:
   (1) Lown-Ganong-Levine (LGL) syndrome is characterized by short PR and normal QRS duration.
   (2) Mahaim-type preexcitation is characterized by normal PR interval and long QRS duration with delta wave.

E. ST Segment and T Wave Changes:
A pathologic ST segment shift assumes either downward slanting followed by diphasic or inverted T wave, or horizontal elevation or depression sustained for longer than 0.08 sec, often accompanied by T wave inversion. Pathologic ST segment shifts are seen in LVH or RVH with "strain," digitalis effect, pericarditis, including postoperative state, myocarditis, myocardial infarction, and some electrolyte disturbances (hypokalemia and hyperkalemia).

1. Pericarditis: ECG changes seen in pericarditis

consist of the following:

a. Pericardial effusion may produce low QRS voltages (QRS voltage <5 mm in every one of the limb leads).
b. Subepicardial myocardial damage produces the following time-dependent changes in the ST segment and T wave:
   (1) ST segment elevation in the leads representing the LV.
   (2) The ST segment shift returns to normal within 2–3 days.
   (3) T wave insertion (with isoelectric ST segment), 2–4 weeks after the onset of pericarditis.

2. Myocarditis: ECG findings of myocarditis (rheumatic or viral) are relatively nonspecific and may include the following changes that involve all phases of the cardiac cycle: first- or second-degree AV block, low QRS voltages (≤5 mm in all six limb leads), decreased amplitude of the T wave, QT prolongation, and arrhythmias or ectopic beats.
3. Myocardial infarction: The ECG findings of myocardial infarction are time dependent and are illustrated in Figure 1–12. Leads that show these abnormalities vary with the location of the infarction and are summarized in Table 1–17.

F. Electrolyte Disturbances:

1. Calcium: *Hypocalcemia* produces prolongation of the ST segment, with resulting prolongation of QTc. The T wave duration remains normal. *Hypercalcemia* shortens the ST segment without affecting the T wave, with resultant shortening of QTc (Fig 1–13).
2. Potassium: *Hypokalemia* produces one of the least specific ECG changes. When the serum potassium K level is below 2.5 mEq/L, ECG changes consist of a prominent U wave (with apparent prolongation of QTc), flat or diphasic T waves, and ST segment depression (Fig 1–14). With

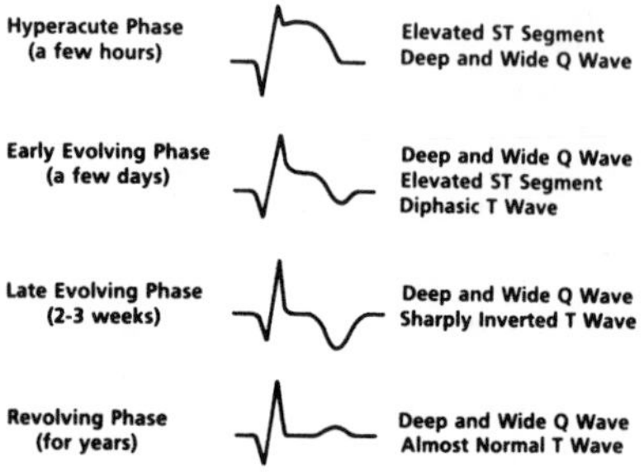

FIG 1–12.
Sequential changes of ST segment and T wave in myocardial infarction. (From Park MK, Guntheroth WG: *How to Read Pediatric ECGs,* ed 2. Chicago, Year Book Medical Publishers, 1987.)

further lowering of serum K, the PR interval becomes prolonged and sinoatrial block may occur. A progressive *hyperkalemia* produces the following ECG changes (see Fig 1–14): (a) tall, tented T waves, best seen in the precordial leads, (b) prolongation of QRS duration, (c) prolongation of PR interval, (d) disappearance of P waves, (e)

TABLE 1–17.
Leads Showing Abnormal ECG Findings in Myocardial Infarction

	Limb Leads	Precordial Leads
Lateral	I, aVL	V5, V6
Anterior		V1, V2, V3
Anterolateral	I, aVL	V2–V6
Diaphragmatic	II, III, aVF	

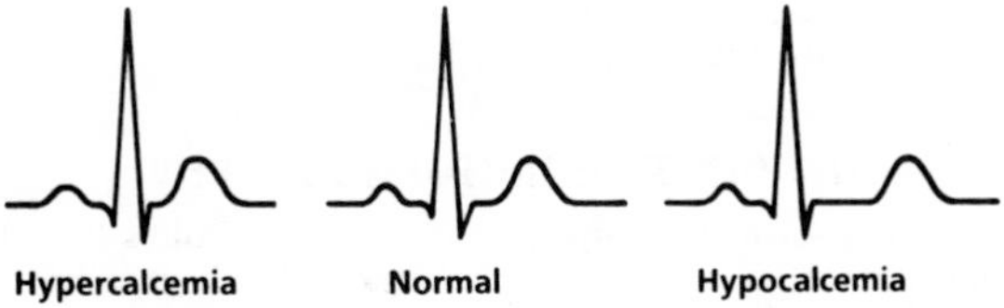

FIG 1–13.
ECG findings of hypercalcemia and hypocalcemia. (From Park MK, Guntheroth WG: *How to Read Pediatric ECGs,* ed 2. Chicago, Year Book Medical Publishers, 1987.)

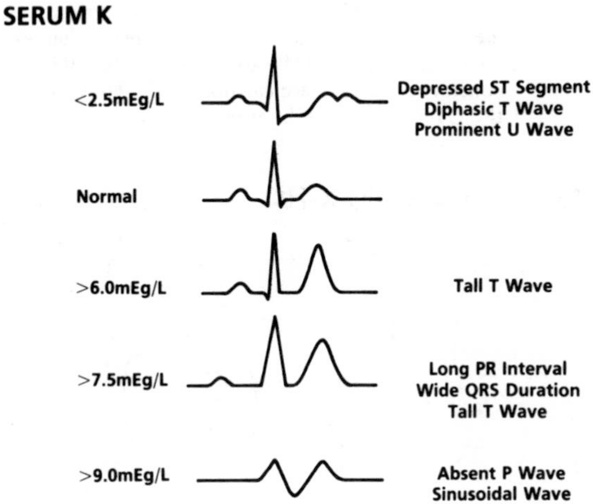

FIG 1–14.
ECG findings of hypokalemia and hyperkalemia. (From Park MK, Guntheroth WG: *How to Read Pediatric ECGs,* ed 2. Chicago, Year Book Medical Publishers, 1987.)

wide, bizarre diphasic QRS çomplexes ("sine wave"), and (f) eventual asystole.

IV. CHEST ROENTGENOGRAPHY

Information to be gained from chest x-ray films (CXR) includes (1) heart size and silhouette, (2) enlargement of specific cardiac chambers, (3) pulmonary blood flow (PBF) or pulmonary vascular markings (PVM), and (4) other information (e.g., lung parenchyma, spine, bony thorax, abdominal situs).

A. Heart Size and Silhouette:

1. Heart size: The cardiothoracic ratio (CT ratio) is obtained by dividing the largest transverse diameter of the heart with the widest internal diameter of the chest. A CT ratio of more than 0.5 is considered to indicate cardiomegaly. However, the CT ratio cannot be used with any accuracy in

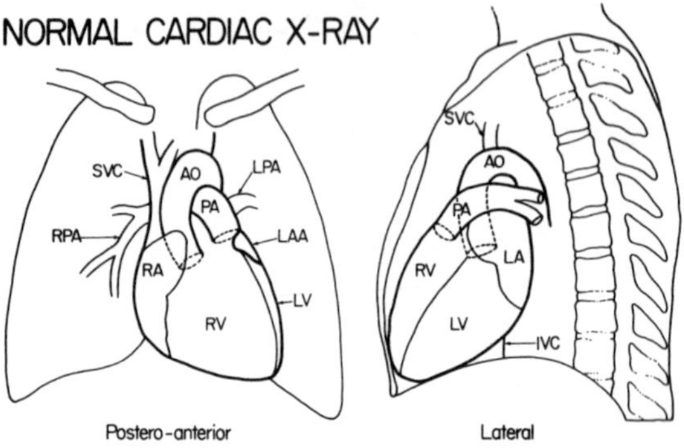

FIG 1–15.
Posteroanterior and lateral projections of normal cardiac silhouette. (From Park MK: *Pediatric Cardiology for Practitioners,* ed 2. Chicago, Year Book Medical Publishers, 1988.)

newborns and small infants, in whom a good inspiratory chest film is rarely obtained.

2. Normal cardiac silhouette: The structures that form the cardiac borders in the PA and lateral projections of a chest roentgenogram are shown in Fig 1–15. In the newborn, however, a typical normal cardiac silhouette as shown in Fig 1–15 is rarely seen because of the presence of a large thymus and because the films are often exposed during expiration.
3. Abnormal cardiac silhouette: The overall shape of the heart sometimes provides important clues to the type of defect, particularly in cyanotic patients (Fig 1–16).
   a. "Boot-shaped" heart with decreased PBF is seen in infants with cyanotic TOF and in some infants with tricuspid atresia.
   b. Narrow waist and "egg-shaped" heart with increased PBF in a cyanotic infant is strongly suggestive of TGA.
   c. "Snowman" sign with increased PBF is seen in infants with the supracardiac type of TAPVR.

B. Cardiac Chambers and Great Arteries:

1. Individual chamber enlargement:
   a. Left atrial enlargement (LAE): Mild LAE is

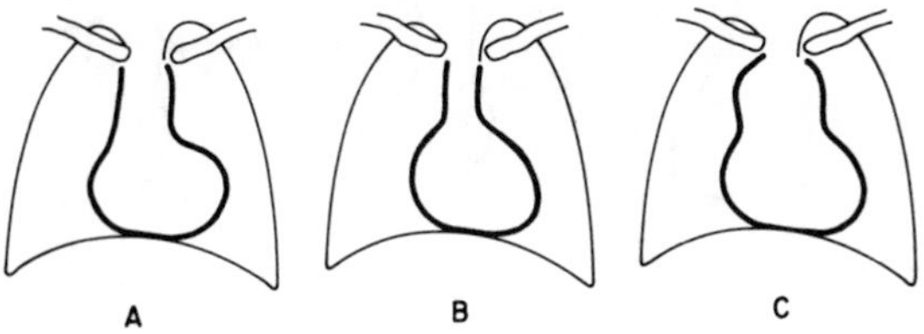

FIG 1–16.
Abnormal cardiac silhouette. **A,** "boot-shaped" heart. **B,** "egg-shaped" heart. **C,** "snowman" sign. (From Park MK: *Pediatric Cardiology for Practitioners,* ed 2. Chicago, Year Book Medical Publishers, 1988.)

best appreciated in the lateral projection by the posterior protrusion of the LA border. An enlargement of the LA may produce "double density" on the PA view. With further enlargement the left atrial appendage becomes prominent on the left cardiac border and the left main stem bronchus is elevated.

b. Left ventricular enlargement (LVE): In the PA view the apex of the heart is displaced to the left and downward. In the lateral view the lower posterior cardiac border is displaced further posteriorly.

c. Right atrial enlargement (RAE): Manifests in the PA projection as an increased prominence of the right lower cardiac silhouette.

d. Right ventricular enlargement (RVE): Best appreciated in the lateral view by the filling of the retrosternal space.

2. Size of the great arteries:

   a. Prominent MPA segment: Prominence of a normally placed pulmonary artery (PA) in the PA view (Fig 1–17,A) is due to one of the following:

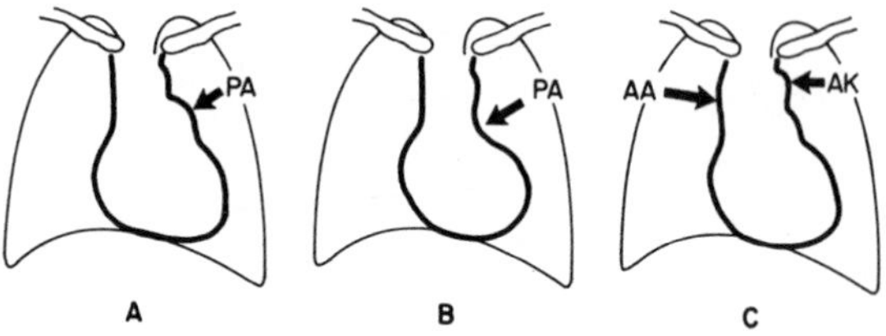

FIG 1–17.
Abnormalities of the great arteries. **A,** prominent main pulmonary artery *(PA)* segment. **B,** concave pulmonary artery segment *(PA)*. **C,** dilatation of the ascending aorta *(AA)* and a prominence of the aortic knob *(AK)*. (From Park MK: *Pediatric Cardiology for Practitioners,* ed 2. Chicago, Year Book Medical Publishers, 1988.)

(1) Poststenotic dilatation (pulmonary valve stenosis).
(2) Increased blood flow through the PA (ASD, VSD).
(3) Increased pressure in the PA (pulmonary hypertension).
(4) Occasional normal adolescence, especially in girls.

b. A concave MPA segment with resulting "boot-shaped" heart is seen in TOF and tricuspid atresia (Fig 1–17,B).

c. Dilatation of the aorta: An enlarged ascending aorta (AA) is seen in TOF and AS (post-stenotic dilatation) and less often in PDA, COA, or systemic hypertension. When the ascending aorta and aortic arch are enlarged, the aortic knob (AK) may become prominent on the PA view (Fig 1–17,C).

C. Pulmonary Vascular Markings (PVM):
One of the major goals of radiologic examination is assessment of the pulmonary vasculature.

1. Increased PVM is present when (a) the pulmonary arteries appear enlarged and extend into the lateral third of the lung field, where they are not usually present, and (b) there is increased vascularity to the lung apices where the vessels are normally collapsed.

   Increased PVM in an acyanotic child represents ASD, VSD, PDA, ECD, PAPVR, or any combination of these. In a cyanotic infant, increased PVM may indicate TGA, TAPVR, HLHS, persistent truncus arteriosus, or single ventricle.

2. Decreased PVM is suspected when the hilum appears small, the remaining lung fields appear black, and the vessels appear small and thin. Ischemic lung fields in cyanotic patients suggest critical stenosis or atresia of the pulmonary or tricuspid valves, and TOF.

3. Pulmonary venous congestion is characterized by

hazy and indistinct margin of the pulmonary vasculature, and is seen with HLHS, MS, TAPVR, and cor triatriatum, for example.

4. Normal pulmonary vasculature is present in patients with mild to moderate obstructive lesions (e.g., PS or AS) and in patients with small L–R shunt lesions.

D. Systematic Approach:

The interpretation of CXRs should include a systematic routine to avoid overlooking important anatomic changes relevant to cardiac diagnosis.

1. Location of the liver and stomach gas bubble: The cardiac apex should be on the same side as the stomach or opposite the hepatic shadow. When there is heterotaxia, with the apex on the right and the stomach on the left, or vice versa, the likelihood of serious heart defect is great. A "midline" liver is associated with asplenia (Ivemark syndrome) or polysplenia syndromes.
2. Skeletal aspect of chest x-ray film: Pectus excavatum may create the false impression of cardiomegaly in the PA projection. Thoracic scoliosis and vertebral abnormalities are frequent findings in cardiac patients. Rib notching is a specific finding of COA in the older child (usually older than 5 years), and is usually found between the fourth and eighth ribs.
3. Identification of the aorta: Right aortic arch is frequently associated with TOF or persistent truncus arteriosus. Precoarctation and postcoarctation dilatation of the aorta may be seen as a "figure-of-3" in a heavily exposed film and as an E-shaped indentation on a barium esophagogram.
4. Upper mediastinum: The thymus is prominent in healthy infants and may give a false impression of cardiomegaly. A narrow mediastinal shadow is seen in TGA and DiGeorge syndrome. "Snowman" sign (figure-of-8 configuration) is seen in infants (usually older than 4 months) with supracardiac TAPVR.

5. Pulmonary parenchyma:
   A long-standing density, particularly in the right lower lung field, suggests bronchopulmonary sequestration. A vertical vascular shadow along the right lower cardiac border may suggest PAPVR from the lower lobe (scimitar syndrome).

V. FLOW DIAGRAM

A flow diagram that often helps in arriving at a diagnosis of CHD is shown in Table 1–18. It is based on the presence or absence of cyanosis and the status of pulmonary blood flow (PBF). Presence of ventricular hypertrophy further narrows the possibilities. Only common entities are listed in the flow diagram.

TABLE 1–18.

Flow Diagram of Congenital Heart Disease

Acyanotic defects	
Increased PBF:	
LVH or CVH:	VSD, PDA, ECD
RVH:	ASD (often RBBB), PAPVR, Eisenmenger's physiology (secondary to VSD, PDA, etc.)
Normal PBF:	
LVH:	AS or AR, COA, endocardial fibroelastosis, MR
RVH:	PS, COA in infants, MS
Cyanotic defects	
Increased PBF:	
LVH or CVH:	Persistent truncus arteriosus, single ventricle, TGA + VSD
RVH:	TGA, TAPVR, HLHS
Decreased PBF:	
CVH:	TGA + PS, Truncus with hypoplastic PA, single ventricle + PS
LVH:	Tricuspid atresia, pulmonary atresia with hypoplastic RV
RVH:	TOF, Eisenmenger's physiology (secondary to ASD, VSD, PDA), Ebstein anomaly (RBBB)

SPECIAL TOOLS IN CARDIAC EVALUATION

II

I. ECHOCARDIOGRAPHY

A. M-Mode Echocardiography (M-mode Echo):
The M-mode Echo, which provides an "ice pick" view of the heart, is important in the evaluation of certain cardiac conditions and functions, particularly in the measurement of dimensions and timing. An M-mode Echo through three important structures of the left side of the heart is illustrated in Figure 2–1.

1. Applications of the M-mode Echo include:
   a. Measurement of the dimensions of cardiac chambers and vessels, thickness of the ventricular septum and free walls.
   b. LV systolic function (fractional shortening, ejection fraction).
   c. Study of the motion of valves (e.g., mitral valve prolapse, MS, pulmonary hypertension) and the interventricular septum.
   d. Detection of pericardial fluid.
2. Normal M-mode echocardiographic values: Normal values of common M-mode Echo measurements according to the weight or BSA of the patient are shown in the Appendix (Tables A–1 and A–3).
3. LV function:
   a. Fractional shortening (FS) of the LV:

$$FS\ (\%) = \frac{Dd - Ds}{Dd} \times 100$$

where Dd = end-diastolic dimension, and Ds = end-systolic dimension. Normal = 36% (28%–44%, 95% CI).

b. Ejection fraction (EF) is obtained by the formula:

$$EF\ (\%) = \frac{(Dd)^3 - (Ds)^3}{(Dd)^3} \times 100$$

Normal = 74% (64%–83%, 95% CI).

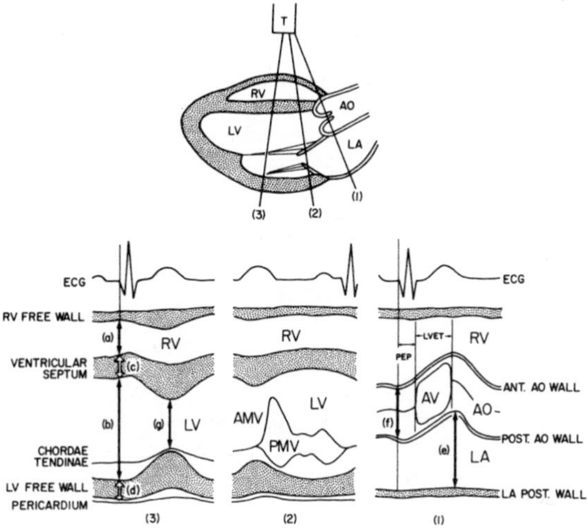

FIG 2–1.

Cross-sectional view of the left side of the heart along the long axis *(top)* through which "ice pick" views of the M-mode Echo recordings are made *(bottom)*. (From Park MK: *Pediatric Cardiology for Practitioners,* ed 2. Chicago, Year Book Medical Publishers, 1988.)

c. Systolic time intervals:
The preejection (PEP) reflects the rate of pressure rise in the ventricle during isovolumic systole. The rate of PEP to the ventricular ejection time (PEP/VET) is little affected by changes in heart rate. The method of measuring LPEP and LVET is shown in Figure 2–1. Normal values (and ranges) for RV and LV are:

$$RPEP/RVET = 0.24\ (0.16\text{–}0.30)$$
$$LPEP/LVET = 0.35\ (0.30\text{–}0.39)$$

B. Two-Dimensional Echocardiography (2D Echo):
The 2D Echo provides enhanced ability to demonstrate the spatial relationship of structures and therefore a more accurate anatomic diagnosis of abnormalities of the heart and great vessels. Routine 2D Echo is obtained from four transducer locations: parasternal, apical, subcostal, and suprasternal notch positions. Figures 2–2 through 2–5 illustrate selected standard images of the heart and great vessels. Selected normal values are presented in the Appendix (Tables A–4 and A–5).

C. Doppler Echocardiography:
Doppler ultrasound equipment detects frequency shifts and thus determines the direction and velocity of blood flow with respect to the ultrasound beam. The pulsed-wave (PW) Doppler has the ability to control the site at which Doppler signals are sampled, but the maximum detectable velocity is limited, and cannot be used for quantification of severe obstruction. On the other hand, continuous-wave (CW) Doppler has the capability of measuring very high velocities for the estimation of severe stenosis.

A positive Doppler indicates a flow toward the transducer, and a negative Doppler a flow away from the transducer. An estimation of pressure gradient ($P_1 - P_2$) can be obtained by a modified Bernoulli equation:

$$P_1 - P_2 = 4\ (V_2^2 - V_1^2) = 4V_2^2$$

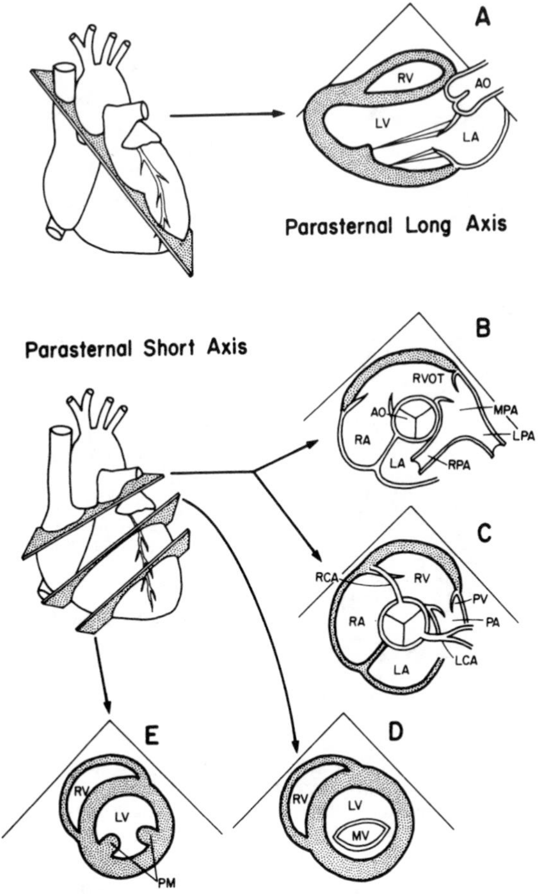

FIG 2–2.
Diagrammatic illustration of important 2D Echo views obtained from the parasternal transducer position. (From Park MK: *Pediatric Cardiology for Practitioners,* ed 2. Chicago, Year Book Medical Publishers, 1988.)

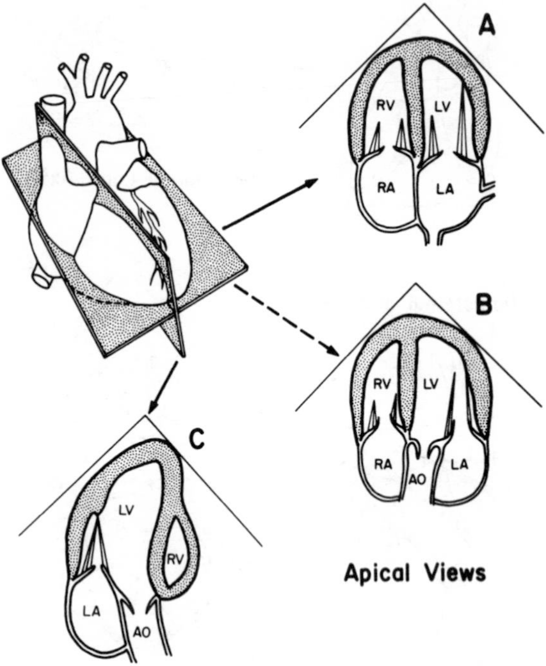

FIG 2–3.
Diagrammatic illustration of 2D Echo views obtained with the transducer at the apical position. (From Park MK: *Pediatric Cardiology for Practitioners,* ed 2. Chicago, Year Book Medical Publishers, 1988.)

where V_2 = peak Doppler velocity beyond the obstruction, and V_1 = peak Doppler velocity proximal to the obstruction. By multiplying the mean velocity of flow and the cross-sectional area, blood flood (cardiac output) can be estimated. Normal Doppler veloc-

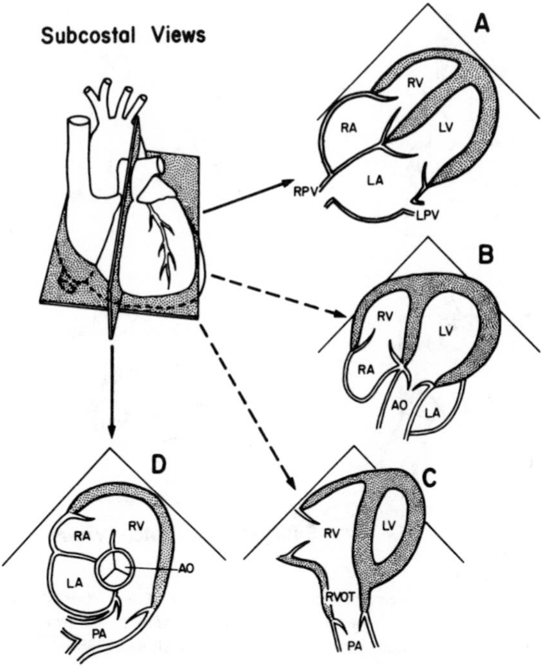

FIG 2–4.
Diagrammatic illustration of 2D Echo views obtained with the transducer at the subcostal position. (From Park MK: *Pediatric Cardiology for Practitioners,* ed 2. Chicago, Year Book Medical Publishers, 1988.)

ities in children (Table A–6) and Doppler Echo formulas (Table A–7) are presented in the Appendix.

D. Color Flow Mapping:
The direction of the flow of blood is shown in red and blue; red denotes flow toward, and blue flow

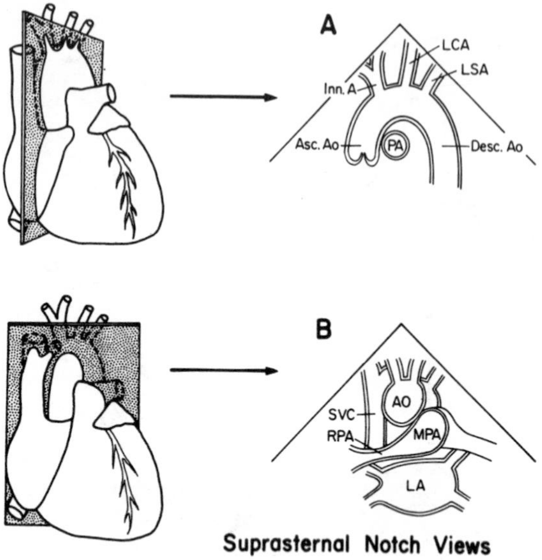

FIG 2–5.
Diagrammatic illustration of 2D Echo views at the suprasternal notch. (Modified from Park MK: *Pediatric Cardiology for Practitioners,* ed 2. Chicago, Year Book Medical Publishers, 1988.)

away from the transducer. A turbulent flow is shown in light green. This is useful in the detection of shunt lesions or valvular lesions.

II. EXERCISE TEST

Exercise testing is important in evaluating cardiac symptoms and arrhythmias, quantifying the severity of cardiac abnormality, and assessing the effectiveness of management. Treadmill protocols are well standardized and more widely used than bicycle ergometer protocols. Normal values for children are now available for the Bruce protocol. Endurance time appears to be the best predictor of exercise capacity in children by the Bruce protocol (Table 2–1).

During stress testing, the patient is continuously monitored for ischemic changes or arrhythmias by ECG, symptoms such as chest pain or faintness, heart rate responses (normal 190–200/min), and blood pressure response (normal systolic pressure may rise to 180 mm Hg).

III. AMBULATORY ELECTROCARDIOGRAPHY

Ambulatory ECGs (Holter monitor) are obtained (1) to document the presence of arrhythmias, (2) to determine the frequency, duration, and types of arrhythmias, (3) to relate symptoms to an arrhythmia, (4) to determine precipitating or terminating events of arrhythmias, (5) to evaluate efficacy of antiarrhythmic agents, and (6) to screen for high-risk cardiac patients (postoperative TGA and TOF).

IV. CARDIAC CATHETERIZATION AND ANGIOCARDIOGRAPHY

Cardiac catheterization and angiocardiography usually constitute the final definitive diagnostic tests for most cardiac patients.

A. Sedation:

These studies are carried out with the patient under general sedation, using various sedatives. A mixture of meperidine (Demerol), chlorpromazine (Thorazine), and promethazine (Phenergan) is widely used. The dose is 0.11 ml/kg of a solution containing 25 mg/ml Demerol, 12.5 mg/ml Phenergan and 12.5 mg/ml Thorazine, with the maximum dose of 2.0 ml IM in infants and older children. Smaller doses (⅓ to ½)

TABLE 2–1.

Bruce Treadmill Test Endurance Times (min)*

	Percentile						
Age (yr)	10	25	50	75	90	Mean	SD
Boys							
4–5	8.1	9.0	10.0	12.0	13.3	10.4	1.9
6–7	9.7	10.0	12.0	12.3	13.5	11.8	1.6
8–9	9.6	10.5	12.4	13.7	16.2	12.6	2.3
10–12	9.9	12.0	12.5	14.0	15.4	12.7	1.9
13–15	11.12	13.0	14.3	16.0	16.1	14.1	1.7
16–18	11.13	12.1	13.6	14.5	15.8	13.5	1.4
Girls							
4–5	7.0	8.0	9.0	11.2	12.3	9.5	1.8
6–7	9.5	9.6	11.4	13.0	13.0	11.2	1.5
8–9	9.9	10.5	11.0	13.0	14.2	11.8	1.6
10–12	10.5	11.3	12.0	13.0	14.6	12.3	1.4
13–15	9.4	10.0	11.5	12.0	13.0	11.1	1.3
16–18	8.1	10.0	10.5	12.0	12.4	10.7	1.4

**Adapted from Cumming GR, Everatt D, Hastman L:* Am J Cardiol *1978; 41:69–75.*

of sedatives are used in infants with cyanosis or CHF. Morphine 0.1 mg/kg SC is used in infants with TOF and possible hypoxic spell. If more sedation is required, IV Valium 0.1 mg/kg or morphine 0.1 mg/kg is used.

B. Normal Hemodynamic Values:

Pressure and oxygen saturation values for normal children are shown in Fig 2–6.

C. Hemodynamic Calculations:

1. Flow (cardiac output) and shunts (by Fick formula):

$$\text{Pulmonary flow (QP)} = \frac{VO_2}{C_{PV} - C_{PA}}$$

$$\text{Systemic flow (QS)} = \frac{VO_2}{C_{AO} - C_{MV}}$$

where flow is given in liters per minute, VO_2 = oxygen consumption (ml/min), C = oxygen con-

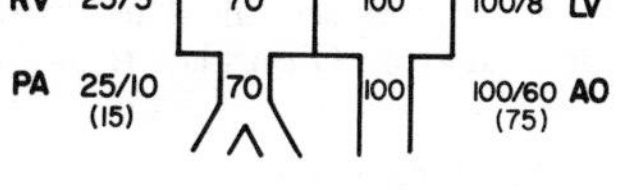

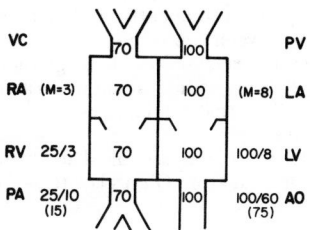

FIG 2–6.
Pressure and oxygen saturation values in normal children.

tent (ml/L) at various positions, PV = pulmonary vein, PA = pulmonary artery, AO = aorta, and MV = mixed systemic venous blood (SVC or RA).

Oxygen consumption is either directly measured during the procedure or estimated from a table (See Table A–8). Oxygen content (ml/100 ml) is derived by multiplying oxygen capacity by percentage saturation. Oxygen capacity (ml/100 ml) refers to the total content of oxygen that hemoglobin contains when it is 100% saturated (1.36 × hemoglobin gm/100 ml). Normal systemic flow (or pulmonary flow in the absence of shunt) is 3.1 ± 0.4 L/min/m^2 (cardiac index).

2. Shunt calculation:
The magnitude of the shunt is calculated as follows:

$$\text{L–R shunt} = Qp - Qs$$
$$\text{R–L shunt} = Qs - Qp$$

In pediatrics the ratio of pulmonary-to-systemic flow (Qp/Qs) is frequently used, and does not require an oxygen consumption value. The ratio provides information on the magnitude of the shunt. Patients with L–R shunt greater than 2:1 are usually surgical candidates.

3. Resistance
Vascular resistances are calculated by using formulas derived from Ohm's law ($R = \Delta P/Q$).

$$\text{PVR} = \frac{\text{Mean PA pressure} - \text{mean LA pressure}}{\text{QP}}$$

$$\text{SVR} = \frac{\text{Mean aortic pressure} - \text{mean RA pressure}}{\text{Qs}}$$

The normal SVR varies between 15 and 30 units/m^2. The normal PVR is high at birth but reaches values near adult values after 2–4 months (1–3 units/m^2). The ratios of PVR/SVR range from 1/20 to 1/10.

D. Selective Angiocardiography:

A radiopaque dye is rapidly injected through a cardiac catheter into a certain site, and angiograms are recorded on motion picture film at 60 or 90 frames per second, often on biplane views. The dose of angiographic dyes for an angiogram ranges from 1 to 2 cc/kg BW, depending on the nature of the defect. Renografin-76 and Hypaque have been commonly used, but a new class of nonionizing contract media (such as ISOVUE-370) is becoming more widely used because of the lower incidence of side effects.

E. Risks:

Cardiac catheterization and angiography can lead to serious complications, including death (rarely), serious arrhythmias, heart block, cardiac perforation, hypoxic spells, arterial obstruction, hemorrhage, infection, reactions to the contrast material, intramyocardial injection of the contrast, and renal complications (e.g., hematuria, proteinuria, oliguria, anuria). Hypothermia, acidemia, hypoglycemia, convulsions, hypotension, and respiratory depression are more likely to occur in the newborn infant.

In general, the risk of cardiac catheterization and angiocardiography varies with the age and illness of the patient, the type of lesion, and the experience of those doing the procedure. The reported rate of fatal complications varies between less than 1% and as much as 5% in the newborn period. About 3% to 5% of patients may have significant but nonfatal complications, such as arrhythmias and arterial complications. However, with more careful preparation and monitoring (see the following discussion) and the use of prostaglandin infusion in selected newborns, the mortality and morbidity can be kept to a minimum.

F. Preparation and Monitoring:

Adequate preparation of the patient before the procedure and careful monitoring during the procedure can minimize complications and fatality from the invasive studies. The following areas are particularly important.

1. Increasing temperature in the cardiac catheterization laboratory when an infant is being examined, and monitoring rectal temperature to avoid hypothermia.
2. Monitoring O_2 saturation transcutaneously; checking arterial blood gases and pH; and correcting acidemia and hypoxemia, and hypoglycemia or hypocalcemia before the start of the procedure.
3. Administering oxygen, if indicated, during the procedure.
4. Intubation or readiness for intubation in infants with respiratory difficulties, and having emergency medications (e.g., atropine, epinephrine, bicarbonate) drawn up and ready.
5. Initiating prostaglandin infusion in cyanotic infants who appear to be ductus dependent.
6. Whenever possible, having another physician or an anesthesiologist available to monitor noncardiac aspects of the patient.

CONGENITAL HEART DEFECTS — III

I. LEFT-TO-RIGHT SHUNT LESIONS

Atrial Septal Defect (Ostium Secundum Defect)

Incidence: 5%–10% of all CHD.

Pathology and Pathophysiology:

1. A defect in the atrial septum may be at the site of fossa ovalis (secundum type), in the lower part of the septum (primum type, or partial ECD), or near the entrance of the SVC or IVC to the RA (sinus venosus type). PAPVR or MVP is occasionally associated with the defect.
2. A L–R shunt is present through the defect with a volume overload to the RA and RV and an increase in PBF. Pulmonary hypertension usually develops in adult life.

Clinical Manifestations:

1. Patients usually have no symptoms.
2. Widely split and fixed S2 and grade 2–3/6 SEM at the ULSB are characteristic. With a large L–R shunt, a mid-diastolic rumble (due to relative TS) may be audible at the LLSB.
3. ECG shows RAD (+90 to +180) and mild RVH or RBBB with rsR′ pattern in V1.
4. CXR shows cardiomegaly (with RAE and RVE), increased PVM, and prominent MPA segment.
5. 2D Echo shows the position as well as the size of the defect.
6. Spontaneous closure of the defect occurs in the first 5 years of life (up to 40% in some series). The defect may decrease in size in some patients. Pulmonary hypertension, CHF, and atrial arrhythmias may occur in adult life (3rd

and 4th decades). Cerebrovascular accident (CVA) due to paradoxical embolization through an ASD is possible.

Management:

Medical: Exercise restriction is not required. SBE prophylaxis is *not* indicated, unless associated MVP or PAPVR is present.

Surgical: Open repair (simple suture or with a patch) under cardiopulmonary bypass (CPB) is performed at the age of 2–5 years, with surgical mortality less than 1%. L–R shunt with Qp/Qs of 2:1 or greater is an indication. Some recommend closure of smaller defects with Qp/Qs <2:1 because of the possibility of a paradoxical embolization resulting in CVA. High PVR ($\geq$10 U/m^2) is a contraindication to surgery.

Ventricular Septal Defect (VSD)

Incidence: Most common form of CHD (20%–25% of all CHD).

Pathology and Pathophysiology:

1. A VSD may be located in the perimembranous septum or in the muscular septum. PDA and COA are frequently associated defects. In subarterial infundibular (or supracristal) VSD, the aortic valve may prolapse through the VSD, with resulting AR.
2. The defect varies in size, ranging from a small defect without hemodynamic significance to a large defect with pulmonary hypertension and CHF. In VSDs with small to moderate L–R shunt, a volume overload is placed on the LA and LV (but not on the RV). With larger defects the RV is under volume and pressure overload in addition to a greater volume overload on the LA and LV. PBF is increased to a varying degree, and pulmonary hypertension may result. With a long-standing large VSD, pulmonary vascular obstructive disease (PVOD)

develops, with severe pulmonary hypertension and cyanosis from a R–L shunt.

Clinical Manifestations:

1. With small VSD, growth and development are normal without symptoms. With moderate to large VSD, decreased exercise tolerance, repeated pulmonary infections, delayed growth and development, and CHF are relatively common in infancy. With PVOD, cyanosis and decreased level of activity may be present.
2. A grade 2–5/6 regurgitant systolic murmur (holosystolic or less than holosystolic) maximally audible at the LLSB is characteristic. A systolic thrill may be present at the LLSB. An apical diastolic rumble is an indication of a large shunt VSD. The S2 may split narrowly, and the intensity of the P2 increases with pulmonary hypertension.
3. ECG: small VSD, normal; moderate VSD, LVH, LAH (±); large VSD, CVH, LAH (±); PVOD, pure RVH.
4. CXR reveals cardiomegaly of varying degree, with enlargement of the LA, LV, and possibly the RV. PVMs are increased. The degree of cardiomegaly and the increase in PVMs are directly related to the magnitude of the L–R shunt. In PVOD the MPA and hilar pulmonary arteries are notably enlarged, but the peripheral lung fields are ischemic.
5. 2D Echo provides accurate diagnosis of the position and the size of the VSD. LA and LV dimensions provide indirect assessment of the magnitude of the shunt. Doppler studies of the PA and the VSD itself can be useful in indirect assessment of RV and PA pressures.
6. Spontaneous closure occurs in 30% to 40% of all VSDs, more frequently in small defects and more often in the first year of life than thereafter. Large defects tend to become smaller

with age. CHF develops in infants with large VSD but usually not until 6–8 weeks of age. PVOD may begin to develop as early as 6–12 months of age in patients with a large VSD, but a R–L shunt usually does not develop until the 2nd decade of life.

Management:

Medical: Treatment of CHF with digitalis and diuretics (see Chapter 7). No exercise restriction is required in the absence of pulmonary hypertension. Maintenance of good dental hygiene and prophylaxis against SBE are necessary.

Surgical:

a. Procedure:
   (1) PA banding as a palliative procedure is rarely performed unless additional lesions make complete repair difficult.
   (2) Direct closure of the defect under CPB and/or deep hypothermia.

b. Indications and timing:
   (1) Significant L–R with Qp/Qs greater than 2:1 is an indication for surgical closure. Surgery is not indicated for a small VSD with Qp/Qs less than 1.5:1.
   (2) Infants with CHF and growth retardation unresponsive to medical therapy should be operated on at any age. Infants with a large VSD and evidence of increasing PVR should be operated on as soon as possible. Those infants who respond to medical therapy may be operated on by the age of 12–18 months. Asymptomatic children may be operated on between 2 and 4 years of age.
   (3) Contraindications: PVR/SVR 0.5 or greater or PVOD with predominant R–L shunt.

c. Surgical approaches for special situations:
   (1) VSD + PDA: If PDA is large, the duc-

tus alone may be closed in the first 6–8 weeks, and the VSD may be closed later.

(2) VSD + COA: Controversies exist. One approach is the repair of COA alone initially without PA banding. The VSD is closed later if indicated.

(3) VSD + AR is usually associated with subarterial infundibular (or supracristal) VSD and occasionally with perimembranous VSD. When AR is present, prompt closure of the VSD is performed, even if the Qp/Qs is less than 2:1, to abort progression of AR or to abolish AR. When AR is moderate or severe the aortic valve is repaired or replaced.

Patent Ductus Arteriosus (PDA)

Incidence: 5%–10% of all CHD, excluding premature infants.

Pathology and Pathophysiology:

1. There is persistent patency of a normal fetal structure between the PA and the descending aorta.
2. The magnitude of the L–R shunt is determined by the diameter and length of the ductus and the level of PVR. With a long-standing large ductus, pulmonary hypertension and PVOD may develop with a R–L shunt and cyanosis.

Clinical Manifestations:

1. Asymptomatic when the ductus is small. When the defect is large, CHF may develop.
2. A grade 1–4/6 continuous ("machinery") murmur best audible at the ULSB or left infraclavicular area is the hallmark of the condition. An apical diastolic rumble is audible with a large shunt PDA. Bounding peripheral pulses with wide pulse pressure are present with large shunt PDAs.

3. ECG findings are similar to those of VSD: normal or LVH in small to moderate PDA, CVH in a large PDA, and RVH in PVOD.
4. CXR findings are also similar to those of VSD: normal with a small-shunt PDA. With a large shunt PDA, cardiomegaly (with LAE, LVE) and increased PVM are present. With PVOD, the heart size is normal, with marked prominence of the MPA and hilar vessels.
5. The PDA can be directly visualized by 2D Echo, and the Doppler examination and color flow mapping in the PA or in the descending aorta confirms the ductal shunt.
6. CHF or recurrent pneumonia develops, if the shunt is large. PVOD may develop if a large PDA with pulmonary hypertension is left untreated.

Management:

Medical: No exercise restriction is required in the absence of pulmonary hypertension. SBE prophylaxis when indicated.

Surgical: Ligation with or without division is indicated for all PDA regardless of size. The presence of PVOD is a contraindication to surgery.

Differential Diagnosis:

The following are the conditions that may present with continuous murmurs.

1. Coronary AV fistula (murmur audible over the precordium, not maximally at the ULSB).
2. Systemic AV fistula (wide pulse pressure with bounding pulse, CHF, and a continuous murmur over the fistula (head or liver) are characteristic).
3. Pulmonary AV fistula (continuous murmur over the back, cyanosis, and clubbing in the absence of cardiomegaly).
4. Venous hum (disappears when the patient is supine).
5. Murmurs of collaterals in patients with COA or TOF.

6. VSD + AR (maximally audible at the MLSB or LLSB and is more to-and-fro than continuous).
7. Absence of pulmonary valve (to-and-fro murmur ("sawing wood" sound) at the ULSB, large central pulmonary arteries on CXR, RVH on ECG, and cyanosis).
8. Persistent truncus arteriosus, occasionally.
9. Aortopulmonary septal defect (AP window).
10. Peripheral PA stenosis (continuous murmur may be audible all over the thorax).
11. Ruptured sinus of Valsalva aneurysm (sudden onset of severe heart failure is characteristic).
12. TAPVR draining into the RA (best audible along the right sternal border).
13. Obstruction to pulmonary venous return following the Mustard operation for TGA (along the right sternal border).

Complete Endocardial Cushion Defect (Complete AV Canal, AV Communis)

Incidence: 2% of all CHD (30% of the defects occur in children with Down's syndrome).

Pathology and Pathophysiology:

1. The complete form of ECD consists of (a) ostium primum ASD, (b) VSD in the inlet portion of the ventricular septum, (c) a cleft in the anterior mitral valve leaflet, and (d) a cleft in the septal leaflet of the tricuspid valve, together with the cleft mitral valve, forming common anterior and posterior cusps of the AV valve. When the ventricular septum is intact, the defect is termed partial ECD or ostium primum ASD.
2. The combination of these defects may result in interatrial or interventricular shunts, LV–RA shunt or AV valve regurgitation. CHF with or without pulmonary hypertension usually develops early in infancy.

Clinical Manifestations:

1. Failure to thrive, repeated respiratory infections, and signs of CHF are common.
2. Hyperactive precordium with a systolic thrill at the LLSB and a loud S2 are frequent findings. A grade 3–4/6 holosystolic regurgitant murmur is audible along the LLSB. The systolic murmur may well be audible at the apex (MR). A mid-diastolic rumble at the LLSB or at the apex (from relative stenosis of tricuspid or mitral valve), and gallop rhythm may be present.
3. ECG finding of left anterior hemiblock ("superior" QRS axis) with the QRS axis between −40 degrees and −150 degrees is characteristic. RVH or RBBB is present in all patients, and many have LVH as well. Prolonged PR interval (first-degree AV block) is common.
4. CXRs always show cardiomegaly with increased PVM.
5. 2D Echo and Doppler with color flow mapping allow visualization of all components of ECD as well as assessment of the severity of the defect.
6. CHF occurs 1–2 months after birth, and recurrent pneumonia is commonly seen. The majority of the patients without surgical intervention die in 2–3 years. The survivors develop PVOD and die in late childhood or young adulthood.

Management:

Medical: Initially, medical management in small infants with CHF, as surgical mortality is relatively high in this age group. SBE prophylaxis is indicated, even on those who have had surgical repair.

Surgical:

a. Palliative: PA banding may be carried out (with a relatively high risk) in small infants if significant MR is not present.
b. Corrective: Closure of ASD and VSD and reconstruction of cleft AV valves under

CPB or deep hypothermia (mortality 5%–10%). Timing varies with institutions and depends on the hemodynamics of the patients (ranges from a few months to several years of age). CHF unresponsive to aggressive medical therapy, repeated pneumonia with failure to thrive, and large L–R shunt with pulmonary hypertension or increasing PVR are indications for surgery.

Partial Endocardial Cushion Defect (Ostium Primum ASD)

Incidence: 1%–2% of all CHD.

Pathology and Pathophysiology: A defect is present in the lower part of the atrial septum near the AV valves. Clefts of the mitral valve and occasionally of the tricuspid valve are present. Pathophysiology is similar to that of ostium secundum ASD.

Clinical Manifestations:

1. Usually asymptomatic during childhood.
2. Findings are identical to those of secundum ASD, with the exception of a regurgitant systolic murmur of MR, which may be present at the apex.
3. ECG shows left anterior hemiblock (or "superior QRS axis"), as in complete ECD. First-degree AV block (50%) and RVH or RBBB (rsR′ pattern in V1) are commonly found.
4. CXR findings are identical to those of secundum ASD, with the exception of LAE and LVE when MR is significant.
5. 2D Echo allows accurate diagnosis of primum ASD by direct visualization of the defect in the lower portion of the atrial septum.
6. CHF may develop in childhood and pulmonary hypertension in adulthood. Infective endocarditis, usually of AV valves, and arrhythmias (20%) may complicate the defect.

Management

Medical: No exercise restriction is required. SBE prophylaxis on indications.

Surgical: Closure of the ASD and reconstruction of the cleft mitral and tricuspid valves under CPB are performed electively at 2–4 years in children with no symptoms or earlier in infants with CHF or MR.

Partial Anomalous Pulmonary Venous Return (PAPVR)

Incidence: Less than 1% of all CHD.

Pathology and Pathophysiology: One or more (but not all) pulmonary veins drain into the RA or its venous tributaries, such as the SVC or IVC, coronary sinus, or left innominate vein. The fundamental hemodynamic alteration is similar to that in ASD.

Clinical Manifestations:

1. Children with PAPVR are usually asymptomatic.
2. Physical findings are similar to those of ASD. When associated with ASD, the S2 is split wide and fixed. When the atrial septum is intact, the S2 is normal.
3. ECG shows RVH or RBBB or may be normal.
4. CXR shows RAE, RVE, and increased PVM.
5. Echo diagnosis of PAPVR is less reliable.
6. Cyanosis and exertional dyspnea may develop during the 3rd and 4th decades due to pulmonary hypertension and PVOD.

Management:

Medical: Exercise restriction is not required. SBE prophylaxis is probably not indicated.

Surgical: Surgical correction is carried out under CPB, usually at the age of 2–5 years. A significant L–R shunt with Qp/Qs greater than 1.5:1 or 2:1 is an indication for surgery, Isolated single lobe anomaly is not ordinarily corrected.

II. OBSTRUCTIVE LESIONS

Pulmonary Stenosis (PS)

Incidence: 5%–8% of CHD.

Pathology and Pathophysiology:

1. Pulmonary stenosis may be valvular (90%), subvalvular (infundibular), or supravalvular. Dysplasia of the pulmonary valve is frequently seen with Noonan's syndrome. Isolated infundibular PS is uncommon, usually associated with a large VSD (TOF).
2. A poststenotic dilatation of the MPA usually develops in valvular PS. Depending on the severity of PS, a varying degree of RVH is present. Dilatation of the RV (on CXRs) does not result unless CHF supervenes.

Clinical Manifestations:

1. Usually asymptomatic with mild PS. Exertional dyspnea and easy fatigability may be seen in moderately severe cases, and CHF in severe cases.
2. A systolic ejection click is present at the ULSB with valvular PS. The S2 may split widely, and the P2 may be diminished in intensity. A systolic ejection murmur (grade 2–5/6) with or without systolic thrill is best audible at the ULSB and transmits fairly well to the back and sides. The louder and longer the murmur the more severe the stenosis.
3. ECG is normal in mild PS. RAD and RVH in moderate PS. RAH and RVH with "strain" in severe PS.
4. Heart size is normal on CXRs, but the MPA segment may be prominent (poststenotic dilatation). PVMs are normal but may be decreased in severe PS.
5. 2D Echo in the parasternal short-axis view may show thick pulmonary valve with restricted systolic motion (doming) and poststenotic dilatation of the MPA. The Doppler study can estimate the pressure gradient.

6. The severity of the obstruction is less likely to progress with age than in AS. CHF and sudden death are possible in more severe PS.

Management:

Medical:

a. Restriction of activity is usually not indicated except for severe PS.
b. Balloon valvuloplasty (performed at the time of cardiac catheterization) is the procedure of choice for significant pulmonary valve stenosis (when systolic pressure gradient is 50 mm Hg or greater).

Surgical:

a. In children with RV pressure greater than 80–100 mm Hg in whom balloon valvuloplasty is unsuccessful, pulmonary valvotomy is performed under CPB or deep hypothermia. Patch widening of the RVOT may be indicated for infundibular PS.
b. Neonates with critical PS may require a transventricular valvotomy while receiving PGE_1 infusion (and left Gore-Tex shunt, if severe infundibular hypoplasia is present).
c. Complete excision of the dysplastic valve with patch widening of the narrowing is done for dysplastic pulmonary valve.

Aortic Stenosis (AS)

Incidence: 5% of all CHD, with male preponderance (male-female ratio = 4:1).

Pathology and Pathophysiology:

1. The stenosis may be valvular, subvalvular, or supravalvular. Valvular stenosis is most commonly due to a bicuspid valve. Supravalvular stenosis is often associated with William's syndrome (mental retardation, characteristic facies, and PA stenosis). Subvalvular stenosis may be due to a simple diaphragm (discrete) or a long, tunnellike narrowing of the LV out-

flow tract. Another type of subvalvular stenosis, idiopathic hypertrophic subaortic stenosis (IHSS), is a primary disorder of the heart muscle.

2. Hypertrophy of the LV may develop, depending on the severity of the stenosis. A poststenotic dilatation of the ascending aorta develops with valvular AS. AR usually develops in subaortic AS.

Clinical Manifestations:

1. Asymptomatic with mild to moderate AS. Exertional chest pain or syncope may occur with severe AS. CHF develops within the first few months of life with critical AS.
2. A systolic thrill is present at the URSB, in the suprasternal notch, or over the carotid arteries. An ejection click may be audible with valvular AS. A rough or harsh SEM (grade 2–4/6) is most audible at the 2RICS or 3LICS, with good transmission to the neck and frequently to the apex. A high-pitched, early diastolic decrescendo murmur (due to AR) may be audible in patients with bicuspid aortic valve and those with (discrete) subvalvular stenosis. Newborn infants with critical AS may develop CHF. The heart murmur may be absent or faint, and the peripheral pulses are weak and thready. The heart murmur becomes louder when CHF improves.
3. A narrow pulse pressure is present in severe AS. A higher systolic pressure in the right arm than in the left arm is found in supravalvular AS.
4. ECG is normal in mild cases. LVH with or without "strain" is seen in more severe cases.
5. CXRs are usually normal in children, but a dilated ascending aorta may be seen occasionally in valvular AS. Significant cardiomegaly does not develop unless CHF develops later in life or unless AR is substantial.

6. 2D Echo may show the anatomy of the aortic valve (bicuspid, tricuspid, or unicuspid) and of subvalvular and supravalvular AS. Doppler examination can estimate pressure gradient in various forms of AS.
7. CHF may develop during the newborn period or later in life with severe AS. Chest pain, syncope, and even sudden death (1%–2%) may occur in children with severe AS.

Management:

Medical:

a. Exercise restriction against sustained strenuous activity is recommended in children with moderate to severe AS. Maintenance of good oral hygiene and SBE prophylaxis when indicated are important.
b. Balloon valvuloplasty may be performed at the time of cardiac catheterization in selected patients. The results are not so promising as for PS.

Surgical:

a. Closed aortic valvotomy using calibrated dilators without CPB may be the procedure of choice in sick infants.
b. Under CPB the following procedures may be performed, depending on the anatomy: (1) aortic valve commissurotomy, (2) replacement with an artificial valve in cases of unicuspid valve, (3) valve replacement following aortic root enlargement (Konno procedure) for severe anular or tunnellike narrowing, (4) excision of the membrane for discrete subvalvular AS, or (5) widening of the stenotic area using a diamond-shaped fabric patch for discrete supravalvular AS.
c. Infants with CHF from critical AS should be operated on at any time. Children with peak systolic pressure gradient of 50–80 mm Hg may be operated on, on an elective

basis. Surgery is indicated in children with symptoms (chest pain, syncope) with "strain" pattern on the ECG or abnormal exercise test, even with systolic pressure gradient slightly less than 50 mm Hg. Earlier elective operation may be considered for subvalvular AS with AR.

Coarctation of the Aorta (COA)

Incidence: 8% of CHD, with a slight male preponderance (male-female ratio = 2:1).

Pathology and Pathophysiology:

1. There is a narrowing of the aorta, most commonly in the upper thoracic aorta. More than 50% of patients with COA have bicuspid aortic valve.
   a. Preductal COA is frequently associated with other cardiac defects (40%), such as VSD, PDA, or TGA. Collateral circulation is poorly developed. These patients become symptomatic very early in life.
   b. Postductal COA is less frequently associated with other cardiac defects and usually does not produce symptoms in infancy.
2. A strong pulse in the arm (frequently with hypertension) and a weak pulse in the leg are characteristic.
3. Preductal COA produces RVH on the ECG in the newborn (rather than LVH, as seen in children). During fetal life the RV is the dominant ventricle that sends blood to the desending aorta and placenta through the ductus arteriosus. With a narrowing proximal to the level of the ductus, the RV ends up handling more blood than does the LV. Therefore, there is a greater degree of RV dominance at birth, with resulting RVH on ECG. This RVH is gradually replaced by LVH by 2 years of age.

I. Asymptomatic Children

Clinical Manifestations:

1. Usually asymptomatic, except for occasional complaints of leg pain.
2. The pulse in the leg is absent or weak and delayed. Hypertension in the arm or higher BP readings in the arm than in the thigh may be present. An ejection click is frequently audible at the apex or at the base. A systolic ejection murmur, grade 2–3/6, is audible at the URSB, MLSB, and in the left interscapular area in the back.
3. ECG usually shows LVH, but it may be normal.
4. CXR shows normal or slightly enlarged heart. An "E sign" on the barium-filled esophagus or "figure-of-3" sign on overpenetrated films may be found. Rib notching may be seen in older children (rarely younger than 5 years of age).
5. 2D Echo may show a discrete shelflike membrane in the posterolateral aspect of the descending aorta. Bicuspid aortic valve is frequently imaged. Doppler examination reveals disturbed flow and increased flow velocity distal to the coarctation.
6. Bicuspid aortic valve may cause stenosis or regurgitation, and LV failure in adult life.

Management:

Medical: Treat hypertension if present. Balloon angioplasty of the COA may be the procedure of choice in selected patients who meet the criteria.

Surgical:

a. Resection of the coarctation segment and end-to-end anastomosis (Fig 3–1,B) is the procedure of choice. Other surgical options are illustrated in Fig 3–1.
b. COA with hypertension in the upper extremities or those with a large pressure gradient between the arms and the legs

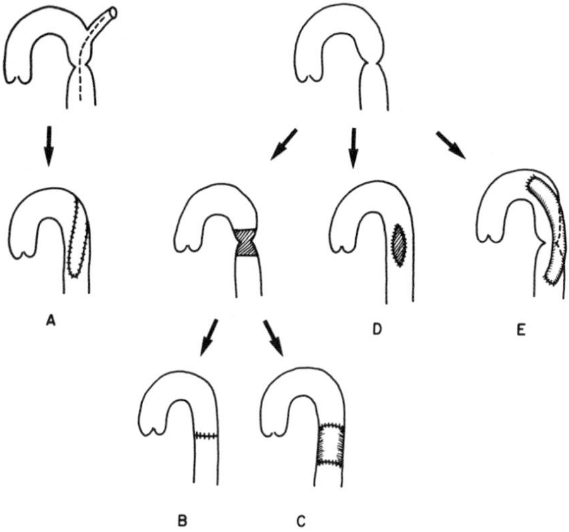

FIG 3–1.
Surgical correction of coarctation of the aorta. (From Park MK: *Pediatric Cardiology for Practitioners,* ed 2. Chicago, Year Book Medical Publishers, 1988.)

should be repaired electively, at age 3–4 years. Children with mild COA (20–30 mm Hg) may be considered for surgery if a prominent pressure gradient develops with exercise.

II. Symptomatic Infants

Clinical Manifestations:

1. Signs of CHF (poor feeding, dyspnea) and renal shutdown (oliguria, anuria) with general circulatory shock may develop in the first 2–6 weeks of life.

2. A loud S3 gallop is usually present, and heart murmur may be absent in sick infants. Weak and thready pulses are present throughout, due to CHF.
3. ECG usually shows RAD and RVH or RBBB (rather than LVH).
4. CXR shows marked cardiomegaly and signs of pulmonary edema or pulmonary venous congestion.
5. 2D Echo shows the site and extent of the COA and other associated defects. The Doppler examination reveals a disturbed flow distal to the COA and signs of a delayed emptying in the aorta proximal to the COA.
6. More than 80% of infants with preductal COA develop CHF by 3 months of age. Early death from CHF and renal shutdown is possible.

Management:

Medical: Intensive anticongestive measures with inotropic agents (catechols), diuretics, and oxygen before surgical treatment. Prostaglandin E1 infusion may be indicated to reopen the ductus arteriosus.

Surgical:

a. If CHF develops, surgery should be performed on an urgent basis. Subclavian flap aortoplasty is preferred by many centers (see Fig 3–1,A). Other surgical options are illustrated in Fig 3–1.
b. If there is a large associated VSD, one of the following procedures may be performed.
   (1) COA repair with no PA banding. If CHF persists, VSD closure is indicated.
   (2) PA banding at the time of COA repair. Later VSD repair and removal of the PA band at 6–24 months of age.

III. CYANOTIC CONGENITAL HEART DEFECTS

Complete Transposition of the Great Arteries (TGA) (D-Transposition, or D-TGA)

Incidence: 5% percent of all CHD; more common in males (male-female ratio = 3:1).

Pathology and Pathophysiology:

1. The aorta arises anteriorly from the RV, and the PA arises posteriorly from the LV. The result is complete separation of the two circuits, with hypoxemic blood circulating in the body and hyperoxemic blood circulating in the pulmonary circuit (Fig 3–2). Defects that permit mixing of the two circulations, such as ASD, VSD, and PDA, are necessary for survival. A VSD is present in 40% of the cases. PS (valvular or subvalvular) occurs in 30%–35% of VSD.
2. In neonates with poor mixing of the two circu-

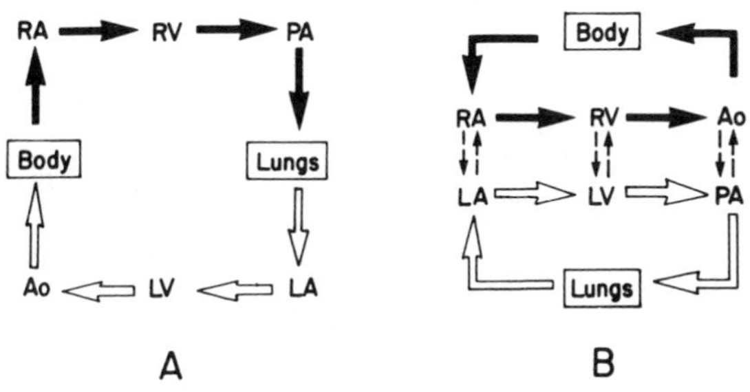

FIG 3–2.
Circulation pathways of normal "in series" circulation **(A)** and "in parallel" circulation of TGA **(B)**. *Open arrows* indicate oxygenated blood, and *closed arrows* desaturated blood. (From Park MK: *Pediatric Cardiology for Practitioners,* ed 2. Chicago, Year Book Medical Publishers, 1988.)

lations, progressive hypoxemia and acidosis develop, with resulting early death. CHF develops in the first week of life in many patients with this condition. The RV is the systemic ventricle, with resulting RVH on ECG.

Clinical Manifestations:

1. Cyanosis and signs of CHF (dyspnea, feeding difficulties) in the newborn period.
2. Auscultatory findings are nonspecific. The S2 is single and loud. No heart murmur is audible in infants with an intact ventricular septum. A systolic murmur of VSD or PS may be present.
3. Severe arterial hypoxemia (unresponsive to O_2 inhalation) and acidosis are present in infants with poor circulation mixing. Hypoglycemia and hypocalcemia are occasionally present.
4. ECG shows RAD and RVH. CVH in infants with large VSD, PDA, PS, or PVOD (as they produce an additional LVH).
5. CXRs show cardiomegaly with increased PVM. An "egg-shaped" cardiac silhouette with a narrow superior mediastinum is characteristic.
6. 2D Echo fails to show a "circle and sausage" of the normal great arteries in the parasternal short axis view; instead, it shows two circular structures. Other views reveal the PA arising from the LV and the aorta arising from the RV. Associated anomalies (VSD, LVOT obstruction, PS, ASD, and PDA) can be visualized.
7. Natural history and prognosis depend on the anatomy.
   a. Infants with an intact ventricular septum are the sickest, but demonstrate the most dramatic improvement following the Rashkind balloon atrial septostomy.
   b. Infants with VSD or large PDA are the least cyanotic, but are most likely to develop CHF and PVOD.
   c. Combination of VSD and PS allows consid-

erably longer survival without surgery but carries a high surgical risk for correction.

d. Cerebrovascular accident and progressive PVOD, particularly in infants with large VSD or PDA, are rare complications.

Management:

Medical:

a. Emergency cardiac catheterization and therapeutic balloon atrial septostomy (Rashkind procedure) are usually performed. PGE_1 infusion may be started to improve arterial Po_2 by reopening the ductus arteriosus.
b. Treatment of CHF with digitalis and diuretics.

Surgical:

a. Palliative procedures: If the Rashkind procedure is unsuccessful in increasing arterial O_2 saturation, a surgical excision of the atrial septum (the Blalock-Hanlon operation) is rarely performed.
b. Definitive repairs: Definitive surgery consists of switching the right- and left-sided structures either at the atrial level (Senning or Mustard operation), at the ventricular level (Rastelli operation), or at the great artery level (Jatene procedure).
    (1) Intra-atrial repair surgeries, especially the Mustard operation, may result in obstruction to the pulmonary or systemic venous return (<5%), tricuspid regurgitation (rare), arrhythmias, and depressed RV function. Sudden death attributable to arrhythmias (3% of survivors) is a rare complication.
    (2) Complications are much fewer with Jatene's operation than with the intra-atrial repair surgeries; pulmonary artery stenosis (<15%) is the only major complication.
    (3) Indication and timing of surgical treat-

TRANSPOSITION OF THE GREAT ARTERIES

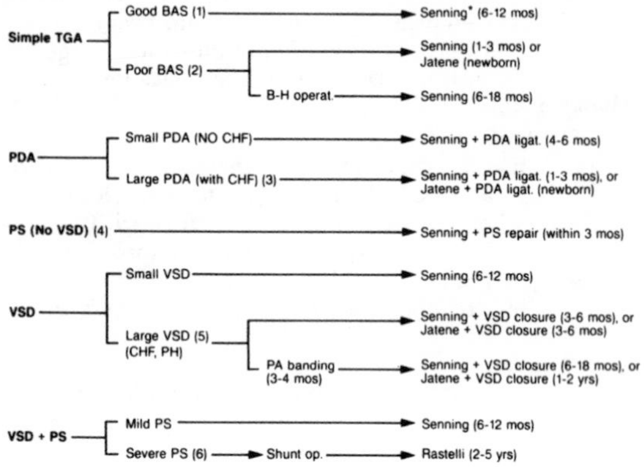

FIG 3–3.
Management flow diagram for TGA. *BAS* = balloon atrial septostomy; *B-H operat.* = Blalock-Hanlon operation; *Senning** is used to represent an intra-atrial repair, either the Senning operation or the Mustard operation. (From Park MK: *Pediatric Cardiology for Practitioners,* ed 2. Chicago, Year Book Medical Publishers, 1988.)

ment vary greatly from institution to institution and are subject to change with the development of new information and new procedures. Fig 3–3 is a partial listing of many approaches used now.

Congenitally Corrected Transposition of the Great Arteries (L-Transposition, L-TGA, Ventricular Inversion)

Incidence: Much less than 1% of all CHD.

Pathology and Pathophysiology:

1. Visceroatrial relationship is normal (RA on the right of the LA). The RA empties into the ana-

tomic LV through the mitral valve, and the LA empties into the RV through the tricuspid valve. For this to occur, the LV is located to the right of the RV (ventricular inversion). The great arteries are transposed, with the aorta arising from the RV and the PA arising from the LV. The aorta is located to the left of and anterior to the PA (L-TGA). The final result is functional correction: oxygenated blood coming into the LA flows to the anatomic RV and out the aorta.

2. Theoretically, no functional abnormalities exist, but most cases are complicated by associated defects, such as VSD (80%) with or without PS, resulting in cyanosis. Systemic AV valve (tricuspid) regurgitation occurs in 30% of patients. Varying degrees of, and sometimes progressive, AV block and paroxysmal SVT are also frequently found.

Clinical Manifestations:

1. Symptomatic during first few months of life with cyanosis (VSD and PS) or CHF (large VSD); asymptomatic when not associated with other defects.
2. The S2 is single and loud. A grade 2–4/6 harsh, holosystolic murmur along the LLSB may indicate VSD or systemic AV valve (tricuspid) regurgitation. A grade 2–3/6 systolic ejection murmur at the ULSB or URSB may indicate the presence of PS.
3. Characteristic ECG findings are the absence of Q waves in leads I, V5, and V6 and/or the presence of Q waves in V4R or V1. Varying degrees of AV block, including complete heart block, may be present. Atrial or ventricular hypertrophy may be present in complicated cases.
4. CXR may show characteristic straight left upper cardiac border (formed by the ascending aorta). Cardiomegaly and increased PVM suggest associated VSD.

5. 2D Echo demonstrates that the RA is connected to the LV and the LV gives rise to the PA or that the LA is connected to the RV and the aorta arises from the RV. Associated cardiac defects can also be identified.

Management:

Medical: Treatment of CHF and arrhythmias, and SBE prophylaxis when indicated.

Surgical:

a. Palliative procedures: PA banding for uncontrollable CHF, and S–P shunt for patients with severe PS.
b. Corrective procedures include closure of VSD (with frequent complication of complete heart block), relief of PS, or valve replacement for significant TR.
c. Pacemaker implantation for complete heart block, either spontaneous or surgically induced.

Tetralogy of Fallot (TOF)

Incidence: 10% of all CHD; most common cyanotic CHD beyond infancy.

Pathology and Pathophysiology:

1. The original description of TOF included four abnormalities: a large VSD, RVOT obstruction, RVH, and overriding of the aorta. However, only two abnormalities are important: a VSD large enough to equalize pressure in both ventricles and an RVOT obstruction. The RVOT may be in the form of infundibular stenosis (50%), pulmonary valve stenosis (10%), or a combination of the two (30%). In the most severe form of the anomaly the pulmonary valve is atretic (10%). Right aortic arch is present in 25% of cases.
2. Because of the nonrestrictive VSD, systolic pressures in the RV and the LV are identical. Depending on the degree of the RVOT obstruction, either an L–R or R–L shunt is

present. With mild PS, an L–R shunt is present ("acyanotic TOF"). With a more severe degree of PS, an R–L shunt occurs (cyanotic TOF). The major heart murmur audible in cyanotic TOF originates from the RVOT obstruction, rather than the VSD.

Clinical Manifestations:

1. Most patients are symptomatic, with cyanosis, clubbing, dyspnea on exertion, squatting, or hypoxic spells. Patients with "acyanotic" TOF are usually asymptomatic.
2. Right ventricular tap and a systolic thrill at the lower and middle LSB are usually found. An ejection click (aortic), a loud and single S2, and a loud (grade 3–5/6) systolic ejection murmur at the middle and upper LSB are present. Occasionally a continuous murmur representing PDA shunt may be audible in a deeply cyanotic neonate (TOF with pulmonary atresia).
3. In the "acyanotic" form, a long systolic murmur resulting from VSD and infundibular stenosis is audible along the entire LSB and cyanosis is absent. (Thus findings resemble those of small-shunt VSD, but the ECG shows RVH or CVH).
4. ECG shows RAD and RVH. CVH may be seen in acyanotic form.
5. In cyanotic TOF, CXR shows normal heart size, decreased PVM, and "boot-shaped" heart with concave MPA segment. Right aortic arch is present in 25% of cases. CXRs of acyanotic TOF are indistinguishable from those of a small to moderate VSD.
6. 2D Echo shows a large VSD and overriding of the aorta. Anatomy of the RVOT and pulmonary valve can be imaged.
7. Children with the acyanotic form of TOF gradually develop the cyanotic form by 1–3 years of age. Hypoxic spells may develop in infants (see below). Brain abscess, CVA, and infective

endocarditis are rare complications. Polycythemia is common, but relative iron-deficiency anemia (hypochromic) with normal hematocrit may result. Coagulopathies are a late complication of long-standing severe cyanosis.

Hypoxic Spell

Hypoxic spells occur in young infants, with peak incidence between 2–4 months of age. It is characterized by (1) a paroxysm of hyperpnea (rapid and deep respiration), (2) irritability and prolonged cry, (3) increasing cyanosis, and (4) decreased intensity of the heart murmur. A severe spell may lead to limpness, convulsion, CVA, or even death.

Pathophysiology of Hypoxic Spell: In TOF, the RV and LV can be considered a single pumping chamber, since there is a large VSD equalizing pressures in both ventricles. Lowering of the systemic vascular resistance (SVR) or increasing resistance at the RVOT can increase the R–L shunting, and this in turn stimulates the respiratory center to produce hyperpnea. Hyperpnea results in an increase in systemic venous return, which in turn increases the R–L shunt through the VSD in the presence of PS. A vicious cycle is established (Fig 3–4).

Treatment of the hypoxic spell is aimed at breaking the vicious cycle. One or more of the following may be useful, in decreasing order of preference:

1. Pick up and hold the infant over the shoulder and place in a knee-chest position.
2. Morphine sulfate, 0.1–0.2 mg/kg SC or IM, suppresses the respiratory center and abolishes hyperpnea.
3. Treat acidosis with $NaHCO_3$ (1 mEq/kg IV). This reduces the respiratory center–stimulating effect of acidosis.

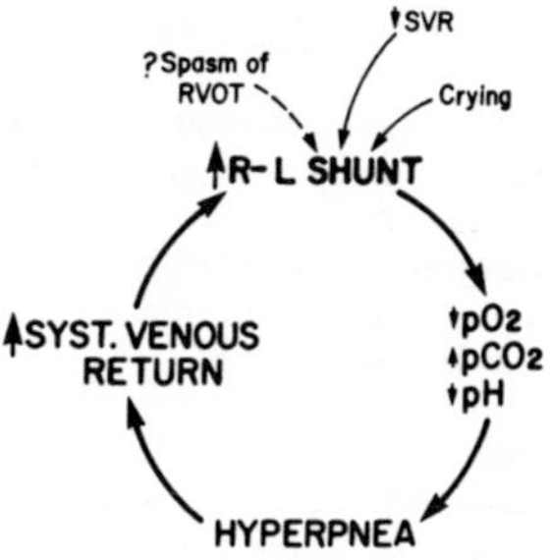

FIG 3–4.
Mechanism of hypoxic spell. (From Park MK: *Pediatric Cardiology for Practitioners,* ed 2. Chicago, Year Book Medical Publishers, 1988.)

4. Oxygen inhalation has limited value, since the problem is reduced PBF, not the ability to oxygenate.

With this treatment, the infant usually becomes less cyanotic and the heart murmur becomes louder, indicating improved PBF. If not fully responsive with the above measures:

5. Vasoconstrictors, such as phenylephrine (Neo-Synephrine) intravenously may be effective. This raises the SVR and forces more blood to the lungs.
6. Propranolol, 2–4 mg/kg/day PO, may be given to prevent hypoxic spells and to delay corrective surgical procedures. The beneficial effect of propranolol may be related to its stabilizing action on peripheral vascular reactivity.

Management:

Medical:

a. Detect and treat relative iron-deficiency anemia. Anemic children are more prone to CVA.

b. Recognize and treat hypoxic spells (see above). Oral propranolol therapy may prevent hypoxic spells.

Surgical:

a. Palliative procedures are indicated to increase PBF in infants with severe cyanosis or uncontrollable hypoxic spells (in whom corrective surgery cannot safely be performed) or in children with hypoplastic PA (in whom the corrective surgery is technically difficult). Different types of systemic-to-pulmonary artery shunt (S–P shunt) have been performed (Fig 3–5).

(1) The Blalock-Taussig shunt (anastomosis between the subclavian artery and the ipsilateral PA) is the procedure of choice in older infants.

(2) Waterston's shunt (anastomosis between the ascending aorta and the right PA) is no longer popular because of many complications following the operation.

(3) Potts operation (anastomosis between the descending aorta and the left PA) is rarely performed.

(4) Gore-Tex interposition shunt between the subclavian artery and the ipsilateral PA (modified B–T shunt) is the procedure of choice in small infants.

b. Conventional Repair Surgery

(1) Symptomatic infants or those with hematocrit 60% or higher who have had no previous shunt procedure and who have favorable anatomy of the RVOT and pulmonary arteries may have primary repair at any time, including in-

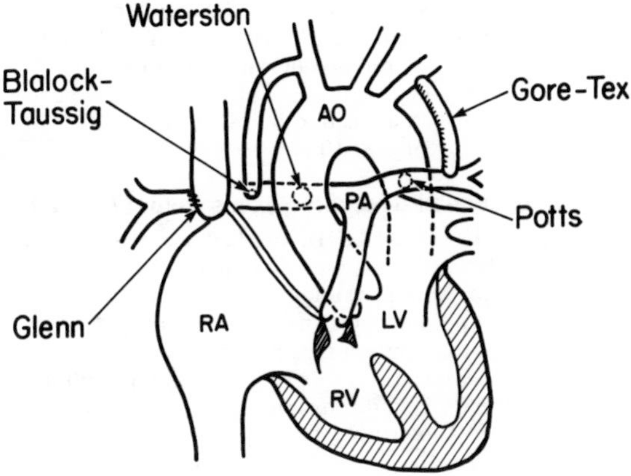

FIG 3–5.
Palliative procedures that can be used in patients with cyanotic cardiac defects with decreased PBF. The Glenn procedure (anastomosis between the SVC and the right PA) may be performed in older infants with hypoplastic RV, as is seen with tricuspid atresia. (From Park MK: *Pediatric Cardiology for Practitioners,* ed 2. Chicago, Year Book Medical Publishers, 1988.)

fancy or even neonatal period. Asymptomatic and minimally cyanotic children who have had previous shunt surgery and children with "acyanotic" TOF may have total repair at 2–4 years of age.

(2) Total repair of the defect is carried out under CPB. The procedure includes patch closure of the VSD and widening of the RVOT by resection of the infundibular tissue, and usually placement of a fabric patch to widen the RVOT.

c. Rastelli's operation is performed when there is severe hypoplasia or atresia of the RVOT.

In this operation the VSD is closed with a patch, and the RV is connected to the PA by an aortic homograft or a valve-bearing prosthetic conduit. This procedure is performed at around 5 years of age, with mortality of 5%–10%.

Total Anomalous Pulmonary Venous Return (TAPVR)

Incidence: 1% of all CHD; marked male preponderance in infracardiac type (male-female ratio = 4:1).

Pathology and Pathophysiology:

1. The pulmonary veins drain into the RA or its venous tributaries, rather than into the LA.
   a. Supracardiac (50%): The common pulmonary vein drains into the SVC, via the left SVC (vertical vein) and the left innominate vein.
   b. Cardiac (20%): The common pulmonary vein drains into the coronary sinus or the pulmonary veins enter the RA separately through four openings.
   c. Infracardiac (subdiaphragmatic) (20%): The common pulmonary vein drains to the portal vein, ductus venosus, hepatic vein, or IVC.
   d. Mixed type (10%): Combination of the above types.

   An interatrial communication (ASD or PFO) is necessary for survival. The left side of the heart is relatively small.
2. Pulmonary venous return reaches the RA, in which systemic venous blood and pulmonary venous blood are completely mixed, before it is shunted to the LA through an ASD. Oxygen saturations in the systemic and pulmonary circulations are the same, resulting in systemic arterial desaturation. The level of systemic arterial oxygen saturation is proportional to the amount of PBF. When there is no obstruction

to pulmonary venous return (seen in the supracardiac and cardiac types), pulmonary venous return is large and the systemic arterial blood is only minimally desaturated. When there is obstruction to pulmonary venous return (seen in the infracardiac type), pulmonary venous return is small and the patient is extremely cyanotic, with signs of pulmonary edema on CXRs.

Clinical Manifestations (without pulmonary venous obstruction):

1. Growth retardation, mild cyanosis, and signs of CHF (tachypnea, dyspnea, tachycardia, hepatomegaly, and growth retardation).
2. Hyperactive RV impulse and characteristic quadruple or quintuple rhythm are present. The S2 is widely split and fixed, and the P2 may be accentuated. A grade 2–3/6 systolic ejection murmur at the ULSB is usually present. A mid-diastolic rumble at the LLSB is always present.
3. ECG shows RAD, RVH of so-called "volume overload" type (rsR′ pattern in V1), and occasional RAH.
4. CXRs show moderate to marked cardiomegaly (involving RA and RV) with increased PVM. A "snowman" sign is seen in older infants (seen rarely before 4 months of age) with the supracardiac type.
5. 2D Echo may visualize the common pulmonary vein posterior to the LA without direct communication to the LA. A markedly dilated coronary sinus protruding into the LA (in TAPVR to the coronary sinus) or dilated left innominate vein and SVC (in the supracardiac type) may be visualized. The obligatory ASD and relatively small LA and LV are visualized.
6. CHF, growth retardation, and repeated pneumonias develop by 6 months of age.

Clinical Manifestations (with pulmonary venous obstruction):

1. Marked cyanosis and respiratory distress are present in the neonatal period.
2. Cardiac findings may be minimal. A loud and single S2 and gallop rhythm are present. Heart murmur is usually absent. Pulmonary rales may be audible.
3. ECG shows RAD and RVH.
4. The heart size is usually normal on CXRs, but the lung fields reveal findings of pulmonary edema.
5. 2D Echo shows relatively hypoplastic LA and LV. Anomalous pulmonary venous return below the diaphragm can also be directly visualized.
6. Patients with the infracardiac type rarely survive more than a few weeks without surgery.

Management (with or without PV obstruction):

Medical:

a. Intensive anticongestive measures with digitalis and diuretics for nonobstructive type.
b. Oxygen and diuretics for pulmonary edema in infants with obstructive type. Intubation and ventilator therapy with oxygen and positive end-expiratory pressure (PEEP) may be necessary in infants with severe pulmonary edema (infracardiac type).
c. Balloon atrial septostomy at the time of cardiac catheterization to enlarge the interatrial communication.

Surgical:

There is no palliative procedure. Corrective surgery is indicated in all patients with this condition; newborns with pulmonary venous obstruction are operated on in the newborn period, and infants without pulmonary venous obstruction by 12 months of age. Procedures vary with the site of the anomalous drainage. The goal is to channel pulmonary venous blood to the LA.

Tricuspid Atresia

Incidence: 1% to 2% of all CHD in infancy.

Pathology and Pathophysiology:

1. The tricuspid valve is absent, and the RV and PA are hypoplastic, with decreased PBF. The great arteries are transposed in 30% of cases. Associated defects, such as ASD, VSD or PDA, are necessary for survival.
2. Systemic venous return is shunted from the RA to the LA, with resulting hypertrophy and enlargement of the RA. The LA and LV are large because they handle both systemic and pulmonary venous return. The degree of cyanosis is proportionally related to the amount of PBF.

Clinical Manifestations:

1. Severe cyanosis, poor feeding, and tachypnea are usual.
2. The S2 is single. A grade 2–3/6 systolic regurgitant murmur (of VSD) at the LLSB is usually present. A continuous murmur (of PDA) is occasionally audible. An apical diastolic murmur may be present with large PBF. Hepatomegaly is present when there is an inadequate interatrial communication or CHF.
3. ECG shows "superior" QRS axis, RAH or CAH, and LVH.
4. CXRs show normal or slightly increased heart size, decreased PVM (increased in infants with TGA), and a "boot-shaped" heart with concave MPA segment.
5. 2D Echo shows absence of a functioning tricuspid valve, large LV and diminutive RV, and ASD. The presence or absence of TGA, VSD, or COA is also shown.
6. Few infants survive beyond 6 months of life without surgical palliation. Occasional patients with increased PBF develop CHF.

Management:

Medical: Treatment of CHF, if present. The Rashkind procedure (balloon atrial septostomy) in small infants as a part of the initial cardiac catheterization to improve the R–L atrial shunt may be needed.

Surgical:

a. Most patients with tricuspid atresia require a palliative procedure to survive. It is to increase PBF (by a shunt operation; see Fig 3–5) when this is deficient and to diminish PBF (by PA banding) when it is excessive.

b. One of the following modifications of the original Fontan operation is performed as definitive surgery:

   (1) Connection of the RA to the PA, either directly or by placement of a conduit, with or without valve.

   (2) Conduit anastomosis of the RA to the RV outflow chamber, with or without valve.

   (3) Anastomosis of each of the divided ends of the SVC to the RPA.

   Infants 4 years of age or older with normal PVR and PA pressure (mean pressure <20 mm Hg), adequate PA size, and normal LV function are good candidates for a Fontan-type operation. Contraindications for the procedure include small or stenotic pulmonary arteries and elevated PVR.

Pulmonary Atresia

Incidence: Less than 1% of all CHD.

Pathology and Pathophysiology:

1. The pulmonary valve is atretic, and the interventricular septum is intact. The RV cavity is usually hypoplastic, with a thick ventricular wall ("peach pit" RV, type I) occurring in about 85% of the cases. Occasionally the RV is

of normal size with significant TR (type II). An interatrial communication (either ASD or PFO) is necessary for survival.

2. Pathophysiologic findings are similar to those of tricuspid atresia. The RA hypertrophies and enlarges to shunt systemic venous return to the LA. The LA and LV handle both systemic and pulmonary venous return and therefore enlarge. PBF depends on the patency of PDA; closure of PDA after birth results in death.

Clinical Manifestations:

1. Severe and progressive cyanosis is present from birth.
2. The S2 is single. Usually no heart murmur is present. A soft, continuous murmur of PDA may be audible at the ULSB.
3. ECG shows normal QRS axis, RAH, and LVH (type I) or occasional RVH (type II).
4. The heart size on CXRs may be normal or large (with RAE). The MPA segment is concave with decreased PVM.
5. 2D Echo usually demonstrates the atretic pulmonary valve and hypoplasia of the RV cavity and tricuspid valve. The atrial communication can be visualized and its size estimated.
6. Prognosis is exceedingly poor without PGE_1 infusion and surgery.

Management:

Medical:

a. PGE_1 (Prostin VR Pediatric solution) infusion as soon as the diagnosis is suspected to maintain patency of the ductus arteriosus during cardiac evaluation and surgery. Starting dosage of Prostin is 0.05–0.1 μg/kg/min; when the desired effect is achieved, reduce the dosage step-by-step, to 0.01 μg/kg/min.

b. A balloon atrial septostomy may be indicated to improve R–L atrial shunt.

Surgical:

a. An S–P shunt (see Fig 3–5) is urgently required, especially for type I. Blind pulmonary valvotomy (Brock's procedure) or transpulmonary valvotomy without CPB is recommended by some at the time of the shunt operation.

b. Follow-up procedures: RVOT reconstruction (placement of patch across the pulmonary annulus) is carried out when the size of the RV is reasonable. For those with hypoplastic RV (type I), the Fontan-type operation may be performed during childhood.

Ebstein's Anomaly

Incidence: Less than 1% of all CHD.

Pathology and Pathophysiology:

1. The leaflets of the tricuspid valve are displaced into the RV cavity; thus a portion of the RV is incorporated into the RA ("atrialized RV") and functional hypoplasia of the RV results. At the same time, tricuspid valve regurgitation results. An interatrial communication is present in the majority (80%) of patients, with resulting R–L atrial shunt.
2. The RA is massively dilated and hypertrophied. In addition, attacks of SVT are frequent, with or without associated WPW syndrome.

Clinical Manifestations:

1. Cyanosis and CHF may develop in the first few days of life. In milder cases, dyspnea, fatigue, and cyanosis on exertion may be present in childhood.
2. The S2 is widely split. Characteristic triple or quadruple rhythm is present (consisting of split S1, S2, S3, or S4). A soft, systolic regurgitant murmur (of TR) is usually audible at the LLSB.
3. Characteristic ECG findings are RBBB and

RAH. WPW syndrome, PAT (SVT), and first-degree AV block are occasionally present.
4. Extreme cardiomegaly (involving principally the RA) and decreased PVM are characteristic x-ray findings.
5. 2D Echo shows the apically displaced septal leaflet of the tricuspid valve.
6. Attacks of PAT (SVT) are common. Other possible complications include CHF, brain abscess, CVA, and infective endocarditis.

Management:

Medical: Anticongestive measures with digitalis and diuretics, if CHF develops. Treatment of PAT with digoxin alone or in combination with propranolol.

Surgical: There is controversy concerning the surgical procedure.

a. Tricuspid annuloplasty is most desirable, although frequently limited by anatomy.
b. Other surgical options include (1) tricuspid valve replacement with a prosthetic or tissue valve and closure of ASD, (2) Glenn's procedure, and (3) a Fontan-type operation.
c. For those patients with WPW syndrome and recurrent PAT, surgical interruption of the accessory pathway is recommended at the time of surgery.

Persistent Truncus Arteriosus

Incidence: Less than 1% of all CHD.

Pathology and Pathophysiology:

1. Only a single arterial trunk (with a truncal valve) leaves the heart and gives rise to the pulmonary, systemic, and coronary circulations. A large VSD is always present. A right aortic arch is present in 50% of patients. Anatomically, this anomaly is divided into four types (Fig 3–6): type I, 60%; type II, 20%; type III, 10%; type IV, 10%.
2. The magnitude of PBF is usually increased in

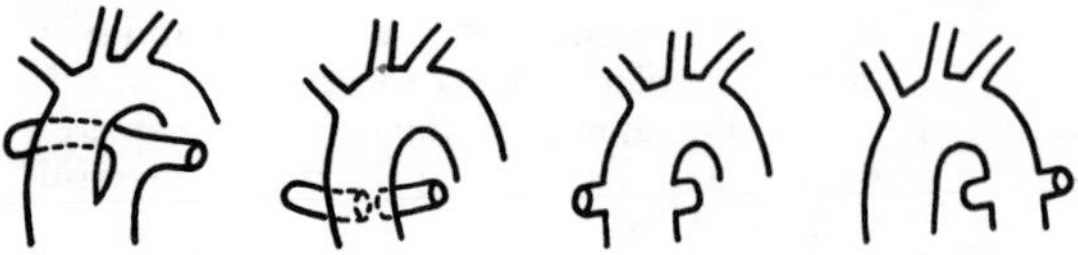

FIG 3-6.
Anatomic types of persistent truncus arteriosus. **A,** type I. **B,** type II. **C,** type III. **D,** type IV, or pseudotruncus arteriosus. (From Park MK: *Pediatric Cardiology for Practitioners,* ed 2. Chicago, Year Book Medical Publishers, 1988.)

type I, normal in types II and III, and decreased in type IV. As with other cyanotic CHDs, the level of systemic oxygen saturation is directly related to the amount of PBF. Therefore, with decreased PBF a notable cyanosis is present. With increased PBF cyanosis is minimal, but CHF may develop. Since there is almost complete mixing of systemic and pulmonary venous blood in the truncus arteriosus, oxygen saturation in the aorta and PA is identical.

Clinical Manifestations:

1. Cyanosis of varying degree may be noted immediately after birth, and signs of CHF develop within several weeks.
2. A harsh (grade 2–4/6) systolic regurgitant murmur (suggestive of VSD) is present along the LSB. An apical diastolic rumble with or without gallop rhythm may be present when PBF is large. Wide pulse pressure and bounding arterial pulses may be present.
3. ECG shows CVH (70%); RVH or LVH is less common.
4. CXRs show marked cardiomegaly (biventricular and LA enlargement) and increased PVM. A right aortic arch is seen in 50% of the cases.

5. 2D Echo demonstrates a large VSD directly under the truncal valve (similar to TOF). The pulmonary valve cannot be shown. A large single great artery arising from the heart (truncus) and the posterior branching of the PA from the truncus may be seen.
6. Most infants die of CHF within 6–12 months without surgery. Clinical improvement occurs if the infant develops PVOD.

Management:

Medical: Vigorous anticongestive measures with digitalis and diuretics are required.

Surgical: PA banding may be indicated in small infants with large PBF and CHF. Rastelli's procedure may be performed for type I or II during infancy. (The VSD is closed in such a way that LV ejects into the truncus, and a valved conduit is placed between the RV and the PA).

Single Ventricle (Common Ventricle, Univentricular Heart)

Incidence: Less than 1% of all CHD.

Pathology and Pathophysiology:

1. Both AV valves empty into a common ventricular chamber. A rudimentary infundibular chamber is usually present and communicates with the common ventricular chamber. A great artery arises from the common chamber, and the other great artery usually arises from the infundibular chamber. TGA is present in 85% of the cases, and AS or PS is common. A high incidence of asplenia or polysplenia syndrome is found.
2. There is a complete mixing of systemic and pulmonary venous blood; therefore oxygen saturation in the aorta and PA is identical. The systemic oxygen saturation is proportional to the amount of PBF. With decreased PBF (seen in patients with associated PS), marked cyanosis

results. In patients without PS, PBF is large and cyanosis is minimal.

Clinical Manifestations:

1. Cyanosis of varying degree is present from birth. Symptoms and signs of CHF, failure to thrive, and bouts of pneumonia are commonly reported.
2. Physical findings are dependent on the magnitude of PBF. With increased PBF, physical findings resemble those of TGA and VSD or even large VSD. With decreased PBF, physical findings resemble those of TOF.
3. ECG:
   a. Unusual ventricular hypertrophy pattern with similar QRS complexes across most or all precordial leads (RS, rS, or QR pattern).
   b. Abnormal Q waves (abnormalities in septal depolarization) are also common and take one of the following forms: (1) Q waves in the RPLs, (2) no Q waves in any precordial leads, or (3) Q waves in both the RPLs and LPLs.
   c. AV block (either first- or second-degree) or arrhythmias (e.g., PAT, wandering pacemaker) may be present.
4. When PBF is increased, CXRs show cardiomegaly and increased PVM. When PBF is normal or decreased, the heart size is normal and the PVM is normal or decreased.
5. 2D Echo shows two distinct AV valves emptying into a single ventricular chamber, and other anomalies (see Pathology and Pathophysiology) are also imaged.

Management:

Medical: Anticongestive measures with digitalis and diuretics.

Surgical:

a. An S–P shunt (in infants) or Glenn's procedure (in children older than 2 years) may be required for patients with PS and severe cyanosis (see Fig 3–5). PA banding in patients without PS and uncontrollable CHF.

b. A modified Fontan procedure may be performed at 4–6 years of age following closure of the tricuspid valve. Mortality is relatively high (20%–30%).

Double-Outlet Right Ventricle (DORV)

Incidence: Less than 1% of all CHD.

Pathology and Pathophysiology:

1. Both the aorta and PA arise side-by-side from the RV. The only outlet from the LV is a large VSD. DORV may be subdivided, depending on the position of the VSD (and further by the presence of PS).
   a. Subaortic VSD (50%–70%) (Fig 3–7,A). PS is common (50%) in this (Fallot) type (Fig 3–7,C).
   b. Subpulmonary VSD (Taussig-Bing anomaly) (Fig 3–7,B).
   c. Doubly committed VSD.
   d. Remote VSD.

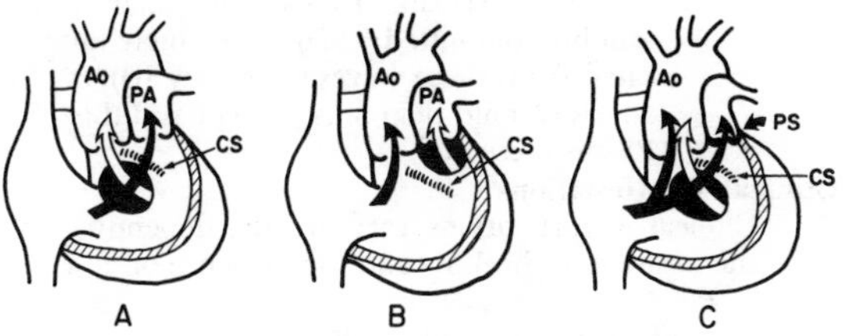

FIG 3–7.

Diagram of three representative types of DORV, viewed with the RV free wall removed. **A,** subaortic VSD. **B,** subpulmonary VSD. **C,** Fallot type. Doubly committed and remote VSDs are not shown. *Open arrow* = oxygenated blood; *solid arrow* = desaturated systemic venous blood. (From Park MK: *Pediatric Cardiology for Practitioners,* ed 2. Chicago, Year Book Medical Publishers, 1988.)

2. Pathophysiology of DORV is determined primarily by the position of the VSD and the presence or absence of PS.
   a. With subaortic VSD, oxygenated blood from the LV is directed to the aorta, and desaturated systemic venous blood to the pulmonary artery, producing mild or no cyanosis (see Fig 3–7,A). The PBF is increased in the absence of PS, resulting in CHF. Therefore clinical findings resemble those of a large VSD with pulmonary hypertension and CHF.
   b. With subpulmonary VSD (Taussig-Bing anomaly), oxygenated blood from the LV is directed to the PA, and desaturated blood from the systemic vein to the aorta, producing severe cyanosis (see Fig 3–7,B). The PBF is increased with the decrease in PVR. Clinical findings therefore resemble those of TGA.
   c. In the presence of PS (Fallot type), clinical findings resemble those of TOF (see Fig 3–7,C).
   d. With the VSD close to both semilunar valves (doubly committed VSD) or remotely located from these valves (remote VSD), cyanosis of mild degree is present and the PBF is increased.

Clinical Manifestations:

Clinical manifestations vary greatly, depending on the location of the VSD and the presence or absence of PS.

1. Subaortic VSD without PS:
   Physical findings resemble those of a large VSD, with pulmonary hypertension and CHF. ECG often resembles that of ECD ("superior" QRS axis, LAH, RVH or CVF and occasional first-degree AV block). CXRs show cardiomegaly with increased PVM and a prominent MPA segment.

2. Subpulmonary VSD (Taussig-Bing malformation):
   Physical findings resemble those of TGA, with severe cyanosis in newborn infants. ECG shows RAD, RAH, and RVH (or LVH during infancy). First-degree AV block is frequently present. CXRs show cardiomegaly with increased PVM.
3. Fallot-type DORV (with PS):
   Physical findings are similar to those seen in cyanotic TOF. ECG shows RAD, RAH and RVH or RBBB. CXRs show normal heart size (with upturned apex) and decreased PVM.
4. Echo (all types of DORV): 2D Echo reveals (1) both great arteries arising from the RV and running a parallel course in their origin, (2) absence of the LVOT, and demonstration of a VSD, and (3) mitral-semilunar discontinuity.

Management:

Medical: Medical treatment of CHF and SBE prophylaxis.

Surgical:

a. Palliative procedures:
   (1) PA banding for symptomatic infants with increased PBF and CHF (subaortic and subpulmonary VSD).
   (2) For infants with Taussig-Bing type, the Blalock-Hanlon operation (atrial septectomy) is essential for better mixing of pulmonary and systemic venous blood.
   (3) S–P shunt procedures in small infants with PS and cyanosis (Fallot type).
b. Corrective surgery:
   (1) Subaortic VSD and doubly committed VSD: Creation of an intraventricular tunnel between the VSD and the root of the aorta.
   (2) Taussig-Bing anomaly (subpulmonary VSD): An intraventricular tunnel between the subpulmonary VSD and

the aorta is most desirable if technically feasible. If not possible, an intraventricular tunnel between the VSD and the PA (converting it to TGA) plus the Jatene (arterial switch) or Senning operation.

(3) Fallot type: An intraventricular tunnel procedure (VSD to Ao) plus relief of PS by patch graft.

(4) Remote VSD: When possible, an intraventricular tunnel procedure (VSD to Ao) is preferred. If not possible, a Fontan-type operation is performed.

IV. MISCELLANEOUS CONGENITAL ANOMALIES

Anomalous Origin of Left Coronary Artery (Bland-White-Garland syndrome)

The left coronary artery arises abnormally from the PA. Symptoms appear at 2–3 months of age and consist of recurring episodes of distress (anginal pain), marked cardiomegaly, and CHF. Significant heart murmur is usually absent. The ECG shows anterolateral myocardial infarction pattern consisting of abnormally deep and wide Q waves, inverted T waves, and ST segment shift in lead I, aVL, and LPLs.

The optimal operation in infancy remains controversial. In the critically ill infant, simple ligation of the anomalous left coronary artery close to its origin from the PA may be carried out to prevent steal into the PA. This should be followed by an elective bypass procedure later. The tunnel operation can be performed in infants who are not critically ill or in those beyond infancy. The tunnel operation consists of creating a 5–6 mm aortopulmonary (AP) window and connecting the opening of the AP window and that of the anomalous coronary artery across the back of the MPA.

Asplenia (Ivemark's) Syndrome

In asplenia syndrome the spleen is absent. Since the spleen is a left-sided organ, bilateral right-sidedness is characteristic. Extremely severe cardiac malformations are always present. Other malformations include two right lungs (three-lobed), midline liver with two gallbladders, malrotation of the gut, and right- or left-sided stomach.

Cardiac malformations include most or some of the following: bilateral SVC, bilateral right atria (with two SA nodes), TAPVR, TGA, pulmonary stenosis or atresia, large ASD or single atrium, ECD, and large VSD or single ventricle. The IVC is commonly on the left side, and azygous continuation is extremely rare.

This syndrome is suggested by midline liver on CXR, superiorly oriented QRS axis in the ECG, varying degree of cyanosis, and the presence of Howell-Jolly and Heinz bodies on blood smear. It is confirmed by a negative radioactive spleen scan. Echo is important in demonstrating various intracardiac anomalies.

The risk of fulminating infection, especially by *Pneumococcus,* is high. Continuous antibiotic therapy in infants up to 2 years of age and immunization with polyvalent pneumococcal vaccine in children 2 years and older are indicated. In patients with decreased PBF, an S–P shunt procedure is indicated. Without a surgical procedure, most patients with asplenia syndrome die in the first year of life (see also Polysplenia Syndrome).

Cor Triatriatum

Cor triatriatum is a rare congenital cardiac anomaly in which the LA is divided into two compartments by an abnormal fibromuscular septum with a small opening, producing obstruction of pulmonary venous return. Hemodynamic abnormalities of this condition are similar to those of mitral stenosis in that both conditions produce pulmonary venous and arterial hypertension.

Important physical findings include dyspnea, basal pulmonary rales, loud P2, and a nonspecific systolic murmur. The ECG shows RAD and severe RVH and occasional

RAH. CXRs show evidence of pulmonary venous congestion or pulmonary edema, prominent MPA segment, and right-sided heart enlargement. Echocardiography demonstrates a linear structure within the LA cavity. Surgical correction is always indicated. Pulmonary hypertension regresses rapidly in survivors if the correction is made early.

Dextrocardia and Mesocardia

The terms "dextrocardia" (heart in the right side of the chest) and "mesocardia" (heart in the midline of the thorax) express the position of the heart as a whole, but do not specify the segmental relationship of the heart.

Segmental Approach

The heart and the great arteries can be viewed as three separate segments: the atria, the ventricles, and the great arteries. These three segments can vary from their normal positions either independently or together, resulting in many possible sets of abnormalities. Accurate chamber localization can be accomplished by Echo and angiocardiography, but CXR and ECG are helpful also.

A. **Localization of Atria:**
   Both CXR and ECG are helpful in localizing the atria.
   1. CXR:
      a. Right-sided liver shadow and left-sided stomach bubble indicate situs solitus of the atria (the RA on the right of the LA, as is normal). Left-sided liver shadow and right-sided stomach bubble indicate situs inversus of the atria (the RA on the left side of the LA).
      b. A midline (symmetric) liver shadow on CXR suggests splenic abnormalities in which either two RA or two LA and other complex cardiac anomalies are present (see Asplenia Syndrome, and Polysplenia Syndrome).
   2. ECG: The SA node is always located in the

RA. Therefore the P axis of the ECG can be used to locate the atria.

a. When the P axis is in the left lower quadrant of the hexaxial reference system (0 to +90 degrees), situs solitus of the atria (RA to the right of the LA) is present.
b. When the P axis is in the right lower quadrant (+90 to 180 degrees), situs inversus of the atria (RA on the left of the LA) is present.
c. With splenic abnormalities, the P axis may be superiorly directed (polysplenia syndrome) or may change between the left lower quadrant and the right lower quadrant from time to time (asplenia syndrome).

B. Localization of Ventricles:

The ECG method of localizing the ventricles is based on the fact that the depolarization of the ventricular septum takes place from the embryonic LV to the RV. This produces Q waves in the precordial leads that lie over the anatomic LV.

a. If Q waves are present in V5 and V6 (as well as lead I) but not in V1, normal relationship of the two ventricles is likely.
b. If Q waves are present in V4R, V1, and V2 but not in V5 and V6, ventricular inversion is likely with the RV located left of the anatomic LV.

C. Localization of Great Arteries:

The ECG is not helpful in localizing the great arteries; however, their location can often be deduced clinically.

Dextrocardia

The four most common types of dextrocardia are classic mirror-image dextrocardia, normal heart displaced to the right side of the chest, congenitally corrected TGA, and single ventricle (Fig 3–8). Less commonly, asplenia and polysplenia syndromes with situs ambiguus and compli-

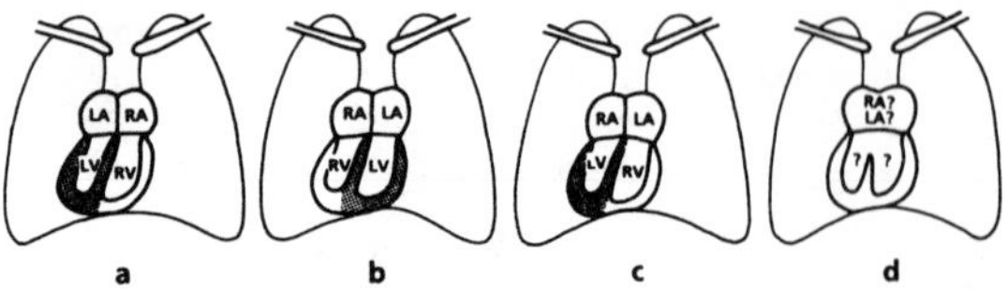

FIG 3–8.
Examples of common conditions when the apex of the heart is in the right side of the chest. (From Park MK, Guntheroth WG: *How to Read Pediatric ECGs,* ed 2. Chicago, Year Book Medical Publishers, 1987.)

cated cardiac defects cause dextrocardia. All of these abnormalities may result in mesocardia.

With CXRs and ECG, the segmental approach discussed above can be used to deduce the nature of segmental relationship in dextrocardia (as well as in mesocardia).

A. In classic mirror-image dextrocardia (see Fig 3–8,A) the liver shadow is on the left on CXRs, and the P axis is between +90 and +180 degrees and Q waves in V5R and V6R on the ECG.
B. With normal heart shifted toward the right side of the chest and the normal R–L relationship maintained (dextroversion) (see Fig 3–8,B), the liver shadow is on the right on CXRs, and the P axis is between 0 and +90 degrees and Q waves in V5 and V6 on the ECG.
C. In congenitally corrected transposition of the great arteries (L-TGA) with situs solitus (see Fig 3–8,C) situs solitus of abdominal viscera is seen on CXRs, and the P axis is in the normal quadrant (0 to +90 degrees) and Q waves in V5R and V6R on the ECG.
D. Undifferentiated cardiac chambers (see Fig 3–8,D) are often associated with complicated cardiac defects and may show midline liver on CXRs. The ECG may show shifting P axis or superiorly ori-

ented P axis and abnormal Q waves in the precordial leads (similar to those described for single ventricle).

Polysplenia Syndrome

Multiple spleens are present in this condition. The spleen is a left-sided organ; therefore bilateral left-sidedness characterizes the syndrome. In addition to cardiac malformations, two left lungs (two-lobed), midline liver, and a right- or left-sided stomach are present.

Cardiac malformations are similar to but less severe than those found in asplenia syndrome. Normal heart is found in occasional patients. Common cardiac malformations include bilateral left atria (with absence of the sinus node), ECD, anomalous pulmonary venous return, and bilateral SVC. The absence of IVC with azygous continuation is characteristic (seen rarely in asplenia syndrome). TGA and DORV are occasional anomalies. Unlike asplenia syndrome, PS is uncommon, and two ventricles are almost always present.

This condition can be suspected by varying degrees of cyanosis, midline liver, and superiorly oriented P axis (due to absence of the sinus node), and superiorly oriented QRS axis (reflecting ECD) on the ECG. The radioactive spleen scan may show multiple splenic tissue.

Although the prognosis is better than that for asplenia syndrome, most infants with severe cardiac malformations die within the first few years of life. An S–P shunt is indicated in those patients with decreased PBF. A greater portion of polysplenia syndrome cases are operable than are asplenia syndrome cases.

Vascular Ring

Vascular ring refers to a group of anomalies of the aortic arch that cause respiratory symptoms or feeding problems. Anatomy, clinical manifestations, and treatment are summarized in Figure 3–9.

Respiratory distress and feeding problems of varying severity appear at various ages. History of pneumonia is frequently elicited. Physical examination is not revealing

	Anatomy	Ba-Esophagogram	Other X-ray Findings	Symptoms	Treatment
Double Aortic Arch	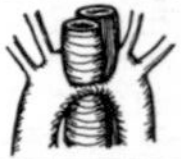	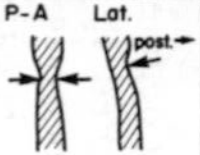	Anterior compression of trachea	Respiratory difficulty (onset < 3 mos.) Swallowing dysfunction	Surgical division of a smaller arch
Right Aortic Arch with Left Lig. Arteriosum	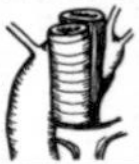	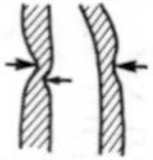		Mild respiratory difficulty (onset > l year) Swallowing dysfunction	Surgical division of the lig. arteriosum
Anomalous Innominate Artery	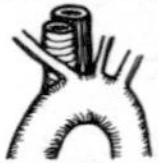	Normal	Anterior compression of trachea	Stridor and/or cough in infancy	Conservative management, or Surgical suturing of the artery to the sternum
Aberrant Right Subclavian Artery	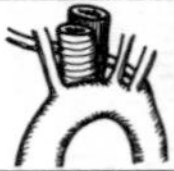	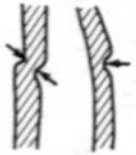		Occasional swallowing dysfunction	Usually no treatment is necessary
"Vascular Sling"	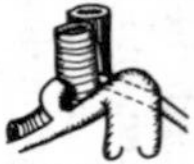	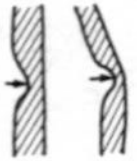	Right-sided emphysema or atelectasis. Posterior compression of trachea or Rt. main-stem bronchus	Wheezing and cyanotic episodes since birth	Surgical division of the anomal. LPA (from the RPA) and anastomosis to the MPA

FIG 3–9.
Summary and clinical features of vascular ring. *P–A* = posteroanterior view; *Lat* = lateral view. (From Park MK: *Pediatric Cardiology for Practitioners,* ed 2. Chicago, Year Book Medical Publishers, 1988.)

except for varying degrees of rhonchi. Cardiac examination and ECG are normal. CXR may reveal compression of the air-filled trachea. Aspiration pneumonia or atelectasis may be present. Barium esophagogram is usually diagnostic, except in anomalous innominate artery (see Fig 3–9). Angiography is usually indicated to confirm the diagnosis and to prepare for surgery.

Medical management is indicated in infants with mild symptoms. A surgical approach is indicated in infants with more severe symptoms or complications such as aspiration pneumonia.

ACQUIRED HEART DISEASE IV

I. PRIMARY MYOCARDIAL DISEASE

Primary myocardial disease is characterized by myocardial insufficiency not associated with any other structural heart disease. Clinically, the majority of these patients have cardiomegaly, signs of CHF, and abnormal ECG.

Endocardial Fibroelastosis (EFE)

Pathology: EFE is a nonobstructive form of primary cardiomyopathy of unknown cause seen in infants and children. The condition is characterized by diffuse changes in the endocardium, with a white, opaque, glistening appearance. The left side of the heart is dilated and hypertrophied, with poor contractility.

Clinical Manifestations:

1. Symptoms and signs of CHF develop in the first 10 months of life.
2. No heart murmur is audible in the majority of patients, although gallop rhythm is usually present. Occasionally a heart murmur of MR is audible. Hepatomegaly is usually present.
3. ECG shows LVH with "strain." Occasionally myocardial infarction patterns and arrhythmias are seen.
4. CXRs show marked cardiomegaly with normal PVM or pulmonary venous congestion patterns.

Treatment: Early and long-term (years) treatment with digoxin, diuretics, and afterload reducing agents is recommended.

Differential Diagnosis: Table 4–1 lists differential diagnosis of cardiomegaly without heart murmur in infants and young children. All of these conditions show

TABLE 4–1.

Differential Diagnosis of Cardiomegaly Without Heart Murmur in Pediatric Patients

- Myocardial diseases
  - Endocardial fibroelastosis (EFE)
  - Myocarditis (viral or idiopathic)
  - Glycogen storage disease
- Coronary artery disease resulting in myocardial insufficiency
  - Anomalous origin of left coronary artery from pulmonary artery
  - Collagen disease (periarteritis nodosa)
  - Kawasaki's disease
- Congenital heart disease with severe heart failure
  - COA in infants
  - Ebstein's anomaly (soft tricuspid regurgitation murmur is frequently present)
- Miscellaneous conditions
  - CHF secondary to respiratory disease (upper airway obstruction, chronic alveolar hypoxia such as seen with BPD, extensive pneumonia)
  - SVT with CHF
  - Pericardial effusion
  - Severe anemia
  - Tumors of the heart
  - Neonatal thyrotoxicosis
  - Malnutrition (infantile beriberi, protein calorie malnutrition)
  - Toxicity (drugs, such as Adriamycin, or radiation)

cardiomegaly on CXR, usually with, but occasionally without, signs of CHF.

Primary Cardiomyopathy

Primary cardiomyopathy, a disease of the heart muscle itself, has been classified into three types based on pathophysiology: hypertrophic, dilated, and restrictive.

A. Hypertrophic Cardiomyopathy:

Pathology: Massive ventricular hypertrophy is present. Although asymmetric septal hypertrophy (ASH), a condition formerly known as idiopathic hypertrophic subaortic stenosis (IHSS), is most common, concentric hypertrophy with symmetric thickening of the LV rarely occurs. Occasionally an intracavitary obstruction may develop during systole, partly because of systolic anterior motion (SAM) of the mitral valve against the hypertrophied septum (hypertrophic obstructive cardiomyopathy, HOCM). The myocardium itself has an enhanced contractile state, but diastolic ventricular filling is impaired because of abnormal stiffness of the LV, which may lead to LAE and pulmonary venous congestion.

Clinical Manifestations:

1. Usually seen in adolescents and young adults, with positive family history in 30% of patients. Easy fatigability, dyspnea, palpitation, or anginal pain may be present.
2. A sharp upstroke of the arterial pulse is characteristic. A late systolic ejection murmur of medium pitch, best audible at the middle and lower LSB or at the apex, is usually heard. A holosystolic murmur of MR is often present. The intensity and even the presence of the heart murmur vary from examination to examination.
3. ECG may show LVH (by voltage criteria), ST-T changes, abnormally deep Q waves (due to septal hypertrophy) with diminished or absent R waves in the LPLs, and arrhythmias.
4. CXRs may show mild LV enlargement with globe-shaped heart.
5. Echo demonstrates an asymmetric septal hypertrophy (ASH) of the interventricular septum. The septum is at least 1.3 times greater than the posterior LV wall. Systolic anterior motion (SAM) of the anterior mitral valve leaflet is also present in the obstructive subgroup.
6. The obstruction may be absent, stable, or slowly progressive. Sudden death may occur, particularly during exercise.

Management:

1. Moderate restriction of physical activity is recommended.

2. A β-adrenergic blocker (e.g., propranolol) is the drug of choice in the obstructive subgroup. Calcium channel blockers (verapamil, nifedipine) may be equally effective. Digitalis, cardiotonic drugs, and vasodilators are contraindicated because they increase the degree of obstruction.
3. Prophylaxis against infective endocarditis is indicated.
4. Transaortic left ventricular septal myotomy and myectomy (Morrow's myectomy) may be indicated in symptomatic patients who are not responding to medical management.

B. Dilated (Congestive) Cardiomyopathy

1. This group is characterized by a weakening of systolic contraction with dilatation of all four cardiac chambers and the development of CHF.
2. Fatigue, weakness, and symptoms of left-sided heart failure (dyspnea on exertion, orthopnea) may be present. A soft systolic murmur (due to MR or TR) with or without gallop rhythm may be audible. Sinus tachycardia, LVH, and ST-T changes are the most common ECG findings. CXRs show generalized cardiomegaly, often with signs of pulmonary venous congestion.
3. Progressive deterioration is the rule rather than the exception. About two thirds of patients die within 4 years after the onset of symptoms, from arrhythmias, embolism, or CHF.
4. Treatment for CHF (e.g., with digoxin, diuretics, bed rest, restriction of activity), anticoagulants (because of the frequency of embolization), and vasodilator therapy (with hydralazine, nitrates, prazosin, or captopril) may prove salutary. Cardiac transplantation may be indicated.

C. Restrictive Cardiomyopathy

1. The least common of the three types is characterized by a restriction to diastolic ventricular filling due to excessively stiff ventricular walls. Contrac-

tile function is unimpaired, thus functionally resembling constrictive pericarditis.
2. History of exercise intolerance, weakness and dyspnea, or chest pain may be present. Jugular venous distention, gallop rhythm, and a systolic murmur of MR or TR may be present.
3. Endomyocardial biopsy may be useful in identifying causes of secondary restrictive cardiomyopathies (e.g., amyloidosis, hemochromatosis, glycogen deposit).
4. Diuretics are beneficial (but digoxin is not indicated, since systolic function is unimpaired). Anticoagulants (warfarin) and antiplatelet drugs (aspirin and dipyridamole) may be used. Corticosteroids and immunosuppressive agents have been suggested.

II. CARDIOVASCULAR INFECTIONS

Subacute Bacterial Endocarditis (SBE; Infective Endocarditis)

Incidence: 0.5–1 per 1,000 hospital admissions, excluding postoperative endocarditis.

Pathogenesis and Pathology:

1. Two factors are important in the pathogenesis of SBE: (a) presence of structural abnormalities of the heart or great arteries with a significant pressure gradient or turbulence (with resulting endothelial damage and platelet-fibrin thrombus formation), and (b) bacteremia, even transient. Bacteremia result frequently from dental procedures and chewing with diseased teeth.
2. All CHD (with the exception of secundum-type ASD) and valvular heart disease predispose to endocarditis. Patients with a prosthetic heart valve or prosthetic material in the heart are at particularly high risk to develop SBE. Drug addicts may de-

velop endocarditis in the absence of known cardiac anomalies.

3. *Streptococcus viridans, Streptococcus faecalis* (enterococcus), and *Staphylococcus aureus* are responsible for more than 90% of cases.

Clinical Manifestations:

1. History of underlying heart defect is present in almost all patients. History of recent dental procedures, tonsillectomy, or toothache is common. Onset is insidious, with fever, fatigue, loss of appetite, and pallor.
2. Heart murmur and fever are almost always present. Splenomegaly is frequently (70%) found.
3. Skin manifestations (50%) are probably secondary to microemboli and may include petechiae, Osler's nodes (tender red nodes at the ends of the fingers), Janeway's lesions (small, painless, hemorrhagic areas on the palms or soles), and splinter hemorrhage (linear hemorrhagic streaks beneath the nails).
4. Embolic phenomena to other organs are present in 50% of cases (e.g., pulmonary emboli, seizures and hemiparesis, hematuria).
5. Carious teeth or periodontal or gingival disease is frequently present.
6. Positive blood cultures, anemia, leukocytosis, and increased ESR are noted.
7. 2D Echo may actually demonstrate the vegetation. It is unlikely that vegetations less than 2 mm in maximum dimension will be seen by 2D Echo.

Diagnosis: A presumptive diagnosis of SBE is made when a patient with an underlying heart lesion has fever of unknown origin of several days duration and any of the above-mentioned physical findings or laboratory changes is present. A definitive diagnosis is made by positive blood cultures. Demonstration of the vegetation by 2D Echo provides a conclusive anatomic diagnosis.

Management:

1. Draw 4–6 blood cultures in succession over 24–48 hours.
2. Start treatment with IV penicillin or oxacillin plus IV gentamicin or IM streptomycin while awaiting the results of blood cultures:
   Penicillin, 6–20 million U/day IV bolus in six divided doses.
   Oxacillin, 200–300 mg/kg/day IV bolus in six divided doses.
   Gentamicin, 7 mg/kg/day IV in three divided doses.
   Streptomycin, 20 mg/kg/day IM in one or two divided doses.
   Final selection of antibiotics depends on the organism isolated and the result of antibiotic sensitivity test. The duration of treatment is 4–6 weeks.
3. Operative intervention may be necessary in patients with prosthetic valves.

Prognosis: Overall recovery rate is 80%–85% (>90% for streptococci and enterococci).

Prevention: Maintenance of good dental hygiene is more important than antibiotic prophylaxis. Provide antibiotic prophylaxis at the time of certain dental or surgical procedures or instrumentation of the upper respiratory, genitourinary, or GI tract, as recommended by the American Heart Association (see Appendix, Fig A–1).

Myocarditis

Etiology: Infection, most commonly by viruses, acute rheumatic fever, some "collagen diseases," or toxic agents, can cause myocarditis.

Clinical Manifestations:

1. History of a URI may be present in older children. There is sudden onset of illness in newborns and small infants, with anorexia, vomiting, and lethargy.

2. Signs of CHF (poor heart tone, tachycardia, gallop rhythm, tachypnea), a soft, systolic heart murmur, and hepatomegaly may be present.
3. ECG shows any one or a combination of the following: low QRS voltages, ST-T changes, prolongation of QT interval, or arrhythmias, especially premature contractions.
4. CXRs always show cardiomegaly of varying degree.
5. Echo reveals cardiac chamber enlargement and impaired LV function.
6. The majority of patients, especially those with mild inflammation, recover completely. Some develop subacute or chronic myocarditis with persistent cardiomegaly with or without signs of CHF, and ECG evidence of LVH or CVH.

Management:

1. Obtain viral cultures from blood, stool, or throat washing and serologic titers.
2. Anticongestive measures include rapid-acting diuretics (furosemide), oxygen, "cardiac chair," and cautious digitalization (using half of the usual dose because some patients may be very sensitive to the drug), or other rapid-acting inotropic agents (isoproterenol or dopamine).
3. The role of corticosteroids is unclear at this time, except for severe rheumatic carditis.

Pericarditis

Etiology:

1. Viral infection is probably the most common cause, particularly in infancy.
2. Acute rheumatic fever is a common cause of pericarditis in certain parts of the world.
3. Bacterial infections (purulent pericarditis), commonly from *S. aureus, Streptococcus pneumoniae, Haemophilus influenzae, Neisseria meningitidis,* and other streptococci.
4. Other causes include tuberculosis (an occasional

cause of constrictive pericarditis), open-heart surgery (postpericardiotomy syndrome), collagen disease, oncologic disease or its therapy, radiation, and uremia (uremic pericarditis).

Pathophysiology:

1. Pathogenesis of symptoms and signs of pericardial effusion is determined by two factors: speed of fluid accumulation and competence of the myocardium. A rapid accumulation of a large amount of fluid or a slow accumulation of a small amount of fluid in the presence of myocarditis can produce circulatory embarassment. Slow accumulation of a large amount of fluid may be well tolerated if the myocardium is intact.
2. With the development of pericardial tamponade, several compensatory mechanisms are called on: (a) systemic and pulmonary venous constriction (to improve diastolic filling), (b) increase in SVR (to raise falling blood pressure), and (c) tachycardia (to improve cardiac output).

Clinical Manifestations:

1. History of URI, precordial pain, and fever may be present.
2. Pericardial friction rub is the cardinal physical sign. The heart is hypodynamic, and heart murmur is usually absent, although it may be present in acute rheumatic fever. In children with purulent pericarditis, septic fever (temperature 101°–105° F), tachycardia, chest pain, and dyspnea are almost always present. Signs of cardiac tamponade may be present (distant heart sounds, tachycardia, pulsus parodoxus, hepatomegaly, venous distention, and occasional hypotension with peripheral vasoconstriction).
3. ECG may show a low voltage QRS complex and ST segment shift and T wave inversion.
4. CXRs may show a varying degree of cardiomegaly. "Water-bottle" shaped heart and increased pulmonary venous markings are seen with large effusion.

5. Echo is the most useful tool in establishing the diagnosis of pericardial effusion and in detecting cardiac tamponade (collapse of the RA or the RV free wall in diastole).

Management:

1. Pericardiocentesis or surgical drainage to identify the cause of the pericarditis is mandatory, especially when purulent pericarditis or tuberculous pericarditis is suspected.
2. Salicylates are indicated for precordial pain from nonbacterial pericarditis and rheumatic fever. Corticosteroid therapy may be indicated in children with severe rheumatic carditis or postpericardiotomy syndrome.
3. For cardiac tamponade, urgent decompression by surgical drainage or pericardiocentesis is indicated. While preparing for pericardial drainage, fluid push with human plasma protein fraction (Plasmanate) to increase central venous pressure is indicated; this helps to improve cardiac filling. Digitalis is contraindicated in cardiac tamponade (because it blocks tachycardia, the compensatory response to impaired venous return).
4. Urgent surgical drainage when purulent pericarditis is suspected. This must be followed by IV antibiotic therapy for 4–6 weeks.

III. KAWASAKI DISEASE (MUCOCUTANEOUS LYMPH NODE SYNDROME)

Etiology: Cause not known. More common in orientals, it is a disease of young children usually younger than 4 years.

Pathology: This generalized febrile illness is accompanied by significant diseases of the heart (vasculitis of the coronary arteries with aneurysm formation), which may be the cause of death. The elevated platelet count seen in this condition contributes to coronary thrombosis.

Clinical Manifestations:

1. Acute phase (first 10 days): Six signs that constitute the diagnostic criteria for Kawasaki's disease (Table 4–2) are present:
2. Subacute phase (11–25 days after the onset) is characterized by:
   a. Desquamation of the tips of fingers and toes.
   b. Significant cardiovascular changes, including coronary aneurysm, pericardial effusion, CHF, or myocardial infarction. ECG shows subtle changes (prolonged PR interval or nonspecific ST-T changes) or abnormal Q waves.
   c. Thrombocytosis (platelet count of 0.6–1 million/mm^3) and elevated ESR are present.
3. Convalescent phase (until elevated ESR and thrombocytosis return to normal): Deep transverse grooves (Beau's line) may appear across each fingernail and toenail.

Natural History and Complications: Self-limited disease in most patients. Cardiovascular involvement is the most serious complication of the disease. Coronary artery aneurysm (25%) is responsible for myocardial infarction (less than 5%) and mortality (1%–2%). Aneurysms have a tendency to regress within 1 year in about 50% of patients.

TABLE 4–2.

Diagnostic Criteria for Kawasaki Disease

1. Fever (temperature spiking to 40° C) persisting for more than 5 days
2. Conjunctival injection (without exudate)
3. Changes in the mouth and lips: strawberry tongue, reddening of oral cavity, and erythema and fissuring of the lips
4. Changes in the hands and feet: reddening of the palms and soles, and indurative edema
5. Erythematous rash
6. Cervical lymphadenopathy (>1.5 cm in diameter)

Diagnosis:

1. Five of six diagnostic criteria are required to make the diagnosis (see Table 4–2). Rule out diseases with similar manifestations (e.g., scarlet fever, Stevens-Johnson syndrome, viral exanthems, sepsis, staphylococcal scalded skin syndrome, Rocky Mountain spotted fever) with appropriate cultures and other laboratory investigations.
2. The possibility of coronary artery involvement should be checked by 2D Echo. Abnormal Q waves in the ECG almost always reflect myocardial damage from coronary artery involvement.

Treatment:

1. Aspirin at high anti-inflammatory dose (100 mg/kg/day) is the treatment of choice. Serum salicylate levels are monitored, and kept near 20 mg/100 mL. When fever subsides the dose is reduced for 2 weeks to 30 mg/kg/day, then to 10 mg/kg/day. Low-dose aspirin therapy is continued for 3 months. Aspirin can be stopped if no aneurysm is identified; but if aneurysm is present aspirin should be continued until the coronary artery appears normal by 2D Echo.
2. High dose γ-globulin (400 mg/kg/day) given IV for 4 consecutive days during the acute phase has been shown to reduce the incidence of coronary artery abnormalities. Corticosteroids are contraindicated because they may increase the incidence of coronary aneurysm.
3. 2D Echo studies are recommended during the acute and subacute phases, and repeated at 3, 6, and 12 months after onset.

IV. ACUTE RHEUMATIC FEVER

Etiology: A delayed sequela of group A hemolytic streptococcal infection of the pharynx (but not of the skin). More common in families with history of rheumatic fever and in those with low socioeconomic status. The peak incidence is at 8 years (range 6–15 years).

Clinical Manifestations:

1. History of streptococcal pharyngitis, 1–5 weeks (average 3 weeks) before the onset of symptoms. The latent period may be as long as 2–6 months (average 4 months) in cases of isolated chorea.
2. Clinical manifestations include some or all findings listed in the revised Jones criteria (Table 4–3), which consist of three groups of important clinical and laboratory findings: five major criteria, five minor criteria, and supporting evidence of preceding streptococcal infection. Diagnosis of acute rheumatic fever is probable when (a) two major criteria or one major plus two minor criteria are present and (b) positive evidence of preceding streptococcal infection is present.
3. Major manifestations:
   a. Arthritis is the most common manifestation (60%–85%) and usually involves large joints (e.g., knees, ankles, elbows, wrists) with characteristic migratory nature. Arthritis subsides in a few days to weeks even without treatment and does not cause permanent damage.

TABLE 4–3.

Jones Criteria (Revised)

Major Manifestations	**Minor Manifestations**
Polyarthritis	Clinical
Carditis	Fever
Chorea	Arthralgia
Erythema marginatum	History of RF or RHD
Subcutaneous nodules	Laboratory
	Acute phase reactants (↑ ESR, +CRP)
	Prolonged PR interval

Plus

Supporting Evidence of Streptococcal Infection

Increased ASO titer

Positive throat culture for group A streptococci

Recent scarlet fever

b. Carditis occurs in 40%–50% of patients. Signs of carditis include some or all of the following:
   (1) Tachycardia (out of proportion for the degree of fever).
   (2) *Significant* heart murmurs (due to MR or AR) are almost always present.
   (3) Pericarditis (friction rub, pericardial effusion, chest pain, and ECG changes).
   (4) Cardiomegaly on CXRs (due to pericarditis, pancarditis, or CHF).
   (5) Signs of CHF (gallop rhythm, distant heart sounds, cardiomegaly).

   Only carditis can cause permanent cardiac damage. Mild carditis disappears rapidly in weeks, whereas severe carditis may last for months.
c. Erythema marginatum (10%) with the characteristic nonpruritic serpiginous or annular erythematous rashes is most prominent on the trunk and the inner proximal portions of the extremities.
d. Subcutaneous nodules (2%–10%) are hard, painless, nonpruritic, freely movable, swelling, 0.2–2.0 cm in diameter. They are usually found symmetrically, singly or in clusters, on the extensor surfaces of both large and small joints, over the scalp, or along the spine.
e. Sydenham's chorea, or St. Vitus' dance (15%), is found more often in prepubertal girls (8–12 years old) than in boys. Emotional lability and personality changes are followed by loss of motor coordination, characteristic spontaneous, purposeless movement, and motor weakness. It is often an isolated manifestation; the patient may have no fever, and ESR and ASO titers may be normal.

4. Minor manifestations include fever, arthralgia, history of rheumatic fever, positive acute phase reactant (↑ ESR, +CRP), and prolonged PR interval (see Table 4–3).

5. Evidence of preceding streptococcal infection. Specific antibody tests are the most reliable laboratory evidence of antecedent streptococcal infection capable of producing acute rheumatic fever. An ASO titer >333 Todd units in children and >250 Todd units in adults is considered significant. Other antibody tests (anti-DNase, anti-NADase, antihyaluronidase, and anti-streptokinase) are less well standardized.

Management:

1. When acute rheumatic fever is suspected, obtain the following laboratory studies: CBC, ESR, CRP, throat culture, ASO titer, CXR, ECG, and possibly Echo.
2. Give benzathine penicillin G, 0.6–1.2 million units IM, for eradication of streptococci and as the first dose of penicillin prophylaxis.
3. Do not start anti-inflammatory or suppressive therapy with salicylates or steroids until definite diagnosis is made.
4. Bed rest is recommended for the duration of the inflammatory process (a few days to 1–2 weeks). The ESR is a helpful guide to the rheumatic activity.
5. Therapy with anti-inflammatory agents should be started as soon as the diagnosis of acute rheumatic fever is made. For minimal carditis or isolated arthritis, aspirin alone, 100 mg/kg/day in four to six doses, is recommended. An adequate blood level of salicylates is 20 mg/100 mL. For moderate to severe carditis, prednisone, 2 mg/kg/day in four divided doses, is indicated. The dose of prednisone should be tapered and aspirin started after 2–4 weeks.
6. Treatment for CHF includes bed rest, oxygen, morphine sulfate, restriction of salt and fluid intake, and furosemide. Digoxin should be used with caution, because certain patients with rheumatic carditis are supersensitive to digitalis; start with half of the usual recommended dose.

7. Management of Sydenham's chorea includes protective measures, elimination of physical and mental stress, and medications such as phenobarbital, chlorpromazine (Thorazine), diazepam (Valium), haloperidol, or steroids.

Prevention:

1. Any patients with documented history of rheumatic fever, including those with isolated chorea and those without evidence of rheumatic heart disease, must receive prophylaxis.
2. Patients should receive prophylaxis until 21–25 years of age. It may be discontinued at that time if the patient (a) has no evidence of valvular involvement and (b) is not in a high-risk occupation (e.g., school teacher, physician, nurse). If the patient has rheumatic valvular disease, prophylaxis is recommended for a longer (possibly indefinite) period.
3. The method of choice for secondary prevention is benzathine penicillin G, 1.2 million units IM every 28 days (not once a month). Alternative methods, although not as effective, include:
   a. Oral penicillin, 200,000–250,000 units twice daily.
   b. Oral sulfadiazine, 0.5 mg once a day for children <60 lb, and 1.0 gm once a day for children >60 lb.
   c. If the patient is allergic to pencillin, erythromycin 250 mg twice daily is recommended.
4. Primary prevention of rheumatic fever is possible with a 10-day course of penicillin therapy for streptococcal pharyngitis.

V. CHRONIC RHEUMATIC HEART DISEASE

Acquired valvular heart diseases are usually of rheumatic origin. Mitral valve involvement occurs in about three fourths and aortic valve involvement in about one fourth of all patients with rheumatic disease. Stenosis and regurgitation of the same valve usually occur together. Isolated

AS of rheumatic origin is extremely rare. Involvement of the tricuspid valve is very rare, and of the pulmonary valve almost never occurs. Therefore only MS, MR, and AR are discussed.

Mitral Stenosis (MS)

Incidence: Although rare in children (since it requires 5–10 years from the initial attack), MS is the most common valvular involvement in adult rheumatic patients.

Clinical Manifestations:

1. Most children with MS are asymptomatic.
2. A narrowly split S2, with accentuated P2 if pulmonary hypertension is present. An opening snap followed by a low-frequency mid-diastolic rumble is audible at the apex. Occasionally a high-frequency diastolic murmur of pulmonary regurgitation (Graham Steell's murmur) is present at the ULSB.
3. ECG may show RAD, RVH, and LAH or CAH. Atrial fibrillation is rare in children.
4. CXRs reveal LAE, RVE, and prominence of the MPA segment. Lung fields may show pulmonary venous congestion, Kerley's B lines, and redistribution of PBF to the upper lobes.
5. M-mode Echo may show large LA dimension, diminished EF slope, and multiple echoes from thickened mitral leaflets. 2D Echo shows doming of thick mitral leaflets and small mitral valve orifice inscribed by the thickened valve. Doppler studies can estimate the valve area.
6. SBE, atrial flutters/fibrillation, and thromboembolism are rare complications in children.

Management:

Medical:

a. Maintenance of good dental hygiene, SBE prophylaxis when indicated, and prevention of recurrence of rheumatic fever with penicillin or sulfonamide. Varying degrees of restriction of activity.

b. Balloon valvuloplasty may delay surgical intervention or result in satisfactory relief of MS.

Surgical:

a. Symptoms (dyspnea on exertion, pulmonary edema, paroxysmal dyspnea), atrial fibrillation, and intractable CHF are indications for surgical approaches.
b. Closed commissurotomy for those with noncalcified valves. Open heart procedures include (1) reconstruction of the valve (valvuloplasty), and (2) artificial valve replacement (in older children with calcified valves and those with combined lesions).

Mitral Regurgitation (MR)

Incidence: The most common valvular involvement in children with rheumatic heart disease.

Clinical Manifestations:

1. Usually asymptomatic during childhood. Rarely, history of fatigue and palpitations.
2. A regurgitant systolic murmur, grade 2–4/6 is present at the apex and often transmits to the left axilla (best demonstrated on left decubitus position). A short, low-frequency diastolic flow rumble may be present at the apex. The S2 may split widely (as a result of shortening of LV ejection and early aortic closure). The S3 is commonly present and loud.
3. ECG is normal in mild MR. LVH or LV dominance is usually present, with occasional LAH.
4. CXRs may show LAE and LVE. PVMs are usually normal, but pulmonary venous congestion pattern may appear if CHF develops.
5. 2D Echo may show dilated LA and LV. Doppler studies detect high-velocity turbulent flows within the LA.
6. Relatively stable for a long time, but MS eventually supervenes in some patients. SBE is a rare complication.

Management:

Medical: SBE prophylaxis and prophylaxis against recurrence of rheumatic fever are indicated. Restriction of activity is not indicated in most mild cases.

Surgical: Indications for surgery include intractable CHF, progressive cardiomegaly with symptoms, and pulmonary hypertension. Valvuloplasty is preferred over valve replacement in children.

Aortic Regurgitation (AR)

Incidence: Most patients have associated mitral valve disease.

Clinical Manifestations:

1. Patients are asymptomatic with mild AR. Decreased exercise tolerance with more severe AR or CHF.
2. A high-pitched diastolic decrescendo murmur, best audible at the 3LICS or 4LICS is present. The longer the murmur the more severe the regurgitation. A systolic ejection murmur of varying intensity may be present at 2RICS. A mid-diastolic mitral rumble (Austin-Flint murmur) is occasionally present. Wide pulse pressure and bounding water hammer pulse develop with severe AR.
3. ECG is normal or shows LVH.
4. CXRs reveal cardiomegaly involving the LV.
5. 2D Echo may show enlargement of the LV. Doppler studies detect a high-velocity diastolic flow into the LV.
6. Patients may be asymptomatic for a long time, but if symptoms begin, many patients deteriorate rapidly. Anginal pain, CHF, or multiple PVCs are unfavorable signs.

Management:

Medical: Maintenance of good dental hygiene, SBE prophylaxis, and prophylaxis against recurrence of rheumatic fever are important. No restriction of activity is indicated for mild cases, but varying degrees of restriction are indicated in more severe cases.

Surgical:

a. Symptoms such as anginal pain and dyspnea on exertion are indications for surgery. Even in asymptomatic patients, significant cardiomegaly, ejection fraction less than 40%, or stress test–induced symptoms may be an indication.
b. Aortic valve replacement under CPB is performed. The antibiotic sterilized aortic homograft appears to be the device of choice.

VI. MITRAL VALVE PROLAPSE (MVP)

Incidence: A reported incidence of 5% in pediatric population is probably an overestimation. More common in adults, with female preponderance (male-female ratio = 1:2).

Pathology: Thick and redundant mitral valve leaflets (due to myxomatous degeneration) bulge into the mitral annulus.

Etiology:

1. Idiopathic in more than 50% of cases. Familial in the primary form (with autosomal dominant mode of inheritance).
2. CHD (30%, most commonly ASD), Marfan's syndrome (nearly all patients), and other connective tissue disorders.

Clinical Manifestations:

1. Although usually asymptomatic, history of nonexertional chest pain, palpitation, and rarely syncope may be elicited.
2. Asthenic build with high incidence (80%) of thoracic skeletal anomalies, such as pectus excavatum, straight back, and scoliosis. Midsystolic click with or without late systolic murmur at the apex is the hallmark of this syndrome. The click may be brought out by held expiration, left decubitus position, sitting, standing, or leaning forward, and may disappear on inspiration.
3. A more specific ECG finding is flat or inverted T waves in leads II, III, and aVF (20%–60%). Ar-

rhythmias (PAT, PAC, PVC), and conduction disturbances (first-degree AV block. WPW syndrome, prolonged QT interval, or RBBB) are occasionally reported.
4. CXRs are usually normal, except for LAE in patients with severe MR.
5. Although results may be false positive or false negative, Echo is usually diagnostic of the condition. 2D Echo is more reliable and shows prolapsing of the mitral valve leaflet(s) superior to the plane of the AV junction, best seen in the parasternal long axis view. Doppler demonstration of MR confirms the diagnosis.
6. The majority of patients are asymptomatic, particularly during childhood. Complications that are rare in childhood include sudden death (from ventricular arrhythmias), SBE, spontaneous rupture of chordae tendineae, progressive MR, CHF, and arrhythmias and conduction disturbances.

Management:

1. Asymptomatic patients require no treatment or restriction of activity. SBE prophylaxis when indicated.
2. Patients with symptoms (palpitation, lightheadedness, dizziness, or syncope) or arrhythmia should undergo ambulatory ECG monitoring or treadmill exercise testing. Propranolol is the drug of choice for ventricular arrhythmias. Chest pain may be treated with propranolol.
3. Reconstructive surgery or mitral valve replacement may be indicated in rare patients with severe MR.

ARRHYTHMIAS AND ATRIOVENTRICULAR CONDUCTION DISTURBANCES

V

The definitions of bradycardia used for adults (fewer than 60/min) and tachycardia (in excess of 100/min) have little significance for children. Tachycardia is present when the heart rate is faster than the upper limit of normal for the patient's age, and bradycardia is present when the heart rate is slower than the lower limit of normal (Table 5–1).

I. BASIC ARRHYTHMIAS

A. Rhythms Originating in Sinus Node

All rhythms that originate in the sinoatrial (SA) node *(sinus rhythm)* have two important characteristics. The five rhythms illustrated in Fig 5–1 all show these characteristics.

a. P waves preceding each QRS complex with a regular PR interval. (The PR interval may be prolonged, as in first-degree AV block).
b. The P axis between 0 degrees and +90 degrees (producing upright P waves in lead II and inverted P waves in aVR).

Regular Sinus Rhythm

The rhythm is regular, and the rate is normal for age; this is normal rhythm at any age.

TABLE 5–1.

Normal Ranges of Resting Heart Rate

Age (yr)	Beats/Min
Newborn	110–150
2	85–125
4	75–115
>6	60–100

Sinus Tachycardia

Description: A rate >140 beats/min in children and >160 beats/min in infants may be significant. The heart rate is usually less than 200 beats/min in sinus tachycardia.

Causes: Anxiety, fever, hypovolemia or circulatory

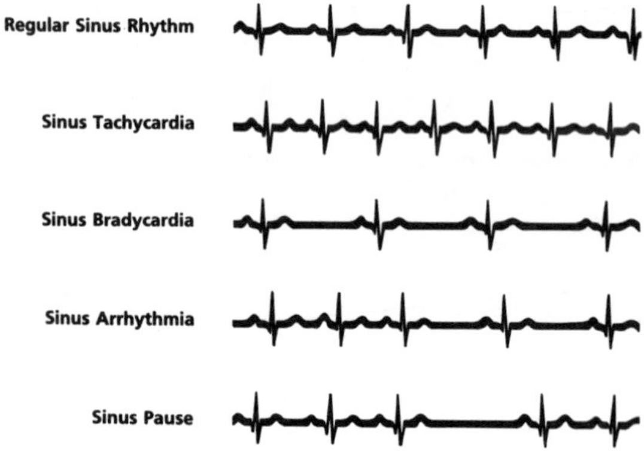

FIG 5–1.

Normal and abnormal rhythms originating in the sinus node. (From Park MK, Guntheroth WG: *How to Read Pediatric ECGs,* ed 2. Chicago, Year Book Medical Publishers, 1987.)

shock, anemia, CHF, catecholamines, thyrotoxicosis, myocardial disease.

Significant: Increased cardiac work is well tolerated by healthy myocardium.

Treatment: Treat underlying cause.

Sinus Bradycardia

Description: A rate <80 beats/min in newborn infants and <60 beats/min in older children may be significant.

Causes: Vagal stimulation, increased intracranial pressure, hypothyroidism, hypothermia, hypoxia, hyperkalemia, and drugs such as digitalis and β-adrenergic blockers; may be normal in athletes.

Significance: In some patients marked bradycardia may not maintain normal cardiac output.

Treatment: Treat underlying cause.

Sinus Arrhythmia

Description: A phasic variation in heart rate, increasing during inspiration and decreasing during expiration.

Causes: A normal phenomenon.

Significance: No hemodynamic significance.

Treatment: No treatment indicated.

Sinus Pause

Description: In *sinus pause* there is momentary cessation of sinus node pacemaker activity, resulting in the absence of P wave and QRS complex for a relatively short duration. *Sinus arrest* is of longer duration and usually results in an escape beat (e.g., nodal escape).

Causes: Increased vagal tone, hypoxia, digitalis toxicity, and sick sinus syndrome.

Significance: No hemodynamic significance.

Treatment: Rarely indicated except in sick sinus syndrome (see following) and digitalis toxicity.

Sick Sinus Syndrome

Description: The sinus node fails to function as the dominant pacemaker of the heart, resulting in a variety of arrhythmias, including profound sinus bradycardia, sinus arrest with junctional escape, paroxysmal atrial tachycardia (PAT), ectopic atrial or nodal rhythm, and bradytachyarrhythmia.

Causes: Extensive cardiac surgery involving the atria (Mustard or Senning procedure), arteritis or focal myocarditis; it is occasionally idiopathic, involving an otherwise normal heart.

Significance: Bradytachyarrhythmia is the most worrisome. Profound bradycardia following a period of tachycardia (overdrive suppression) can cause syncope and even death.

Treatment: Antiarrhythmic drugs, such as propranolol or quinidine, are indicated to suppress tachycardia. Demand ventricular pacemaker may be required for symptomatic patients with episodes of extreme bradycardia.

B. Rhythms Originating in Atrium (Ectopic Atrial Rhythm)

Atrial arrhythmias are characterized by the following (Fig 5–2):

a. P waves of unusual contour (abnormal P axis), and/or abnormal number of P waves per QRS complex, and
b. QRS complexes of normal duration (but with occasional wide QRS duration [aberrancy]).

Premature Atrial Contraction (PAC)

Description: The QRS complex occurs prematurely, with abnormal P wave morphology. There is an incomplete compensatory pause: the length of two cycles, including one premature beat, is less than the length of two normal cycles. Occasional PACs are not followed by QRS complex (nonconducted PAC) (see Fig 5–2).

Causes: Seen in healthy children, including the newborn, after cardiac surgery; digitalis toxicity.

Significance: No hemodynamic significance.

Treatment: Usually no treatment indicated, except in digitalis toxicity.

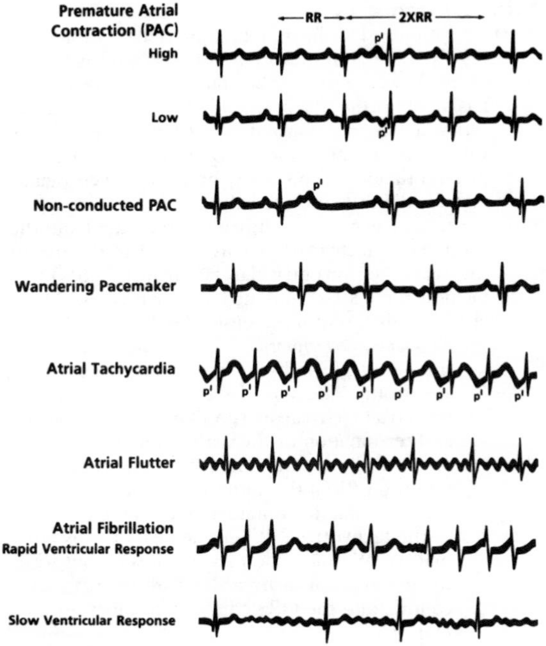

FIG 5–2.
Arrhythmias originating in the atrium. (From Park MK, Guntheroth WG: *How to Read Pediatric ECGs*, ed 2. Chicago, Year Book Medical Publishers, 1987.)

Wandering Atrial Pacemaker

Description: Gradual changes in the shape of P waves and PR intervals. QRS complex is normal.
Causes: Seen in otherwise healthy children.
Significance: No clinical significance.
Treatment: No treatment indicated.

Atrial Tachycardia

Description: The heart rate is extremely rapid and regular (240 ± 40 beats/min). The P wave is buried in the T wave and invisible, but when visible usually has an abnormal P axis (see Fig 5–2). The QRS duration is usually normal. Occasionally, aberrancy will cause prolongation of QRS duration, making differentiation of this arrhythmia from ventricular tachycardia difficult (see below).

Atrial tachycardia is difficult to separate from the rarer nodal tachycardia. This has led to the use of the term "supraventricular tachycardia" (SVT) to include both atrial and nodal tachycardias. There are three different mechanisms for SVT:

a. *AV reentry or reciprocating tachycardia* is the most common tachyarrhythmia seen in the pediatric age group. This was formerly called paroxysmal atrial tachycardia (PAT) because the onset and termination of this arrhythmia were characteristically abrupt. The retrograde conduction (of a PVC) through the bundle of Kent is responsible for initiation and maintenance of the tachycardia. When the heart rate is normal, WPW syndrome may be present, but with the initiation of tachycardia (with retrograde conduction) the QRS complex becomes normal.
b. *Ectopic or nonreciprocating atrial tachycardia* is a rare mechanism of SVT, in which rapid firing of a single focus in the atrium is responsible for the tachycardia. Unlike reciprocating atrial tachycardia, in ectopic atrial tachycardia the heart rate may vary substantially during the course of a day and second-degree AV block may develop.
c. *Nodal tachycardia* may superficially resemble atrial tachycardia, but the rate of nodal tachycardia is relatively slower (120–200 beats/min) than atrial tachycardia.

Causes:

a. Idiopathic type (50%) occurs more commonly in young infants than in older children.
b. WPW syndrome (10% – 20%) and CHD (Ebstein's anomaly, single ventricle, L-TGA).

Significance: May decrease cardiac output and result in CHF, with rapid deterioration.

Treatment:

a. Vagal stimulatory maneuvers (carotid sinus massage, gagging, pressure on eyeball) may be effective in older children but are rarely effective in infants
b. Placing an icebag on the face (up to 10 sec) is often successful in infants.
c. Initial cardioversion may be performed in infants with signs of CHF and those with wide QRS complexes in which differentiation between ventricular tachycardia and atrial tachycardia with an aberrancy is difficult. The initial dose of 0.5 w·sec/kg may be increased step-by-step to 2 w·sec/kg. This is followed by digitalization.
d. Digitalization is the method of choice in infants without CHF and those with mild CHF.
e. If the patient is not in CHF and digitalis is not effective, IV infusion of phenylephrine may be tried (not recommended in patients with CHF). It raises blood pressure abruptly and converts the tachycardia by reflex increase in vagal tone.
f. IV administration of propranolol or verapamil may be tried but is certainly not the treatment of choice. These drugs may produce extreme bradycardia and hypotension in infants younger than 1 year of age and should be avoided when possible.
g. Overdrive suppression by atrial or esophageal pacing may be indicated in children who are already digitalized. Cardioversion carries a risk of inducing ventricular tachycardia in digi-

talized patients. Transesophageal pacing has been shown to be safe and effective.

h. Prevention of recurrence of PAT with maintenance dosage of digoxin for 3–6 months is recommended. In patients with WPW syndrome propranolol may be effective in preventing further attacks. In occasional patients with WPW syndrome surgical interruption of accessory pathways should be considered if medical management fails.

Atrial Flutter

Description: Characterized by a fast atrial rate ("F" wave with "sawtooth" configuration) of about 300 beats/min, the ventricle responding with varying degrees of block (e.g., 2:1, 3:1, 4:1) and normal QRS complexes (see Fig 5–2).

Causes: Structural heart disease with dilated atria, myocarditis, previous surgery involving atria (Mustard procedure or ASD repair), or digitalis toxicity.

Significance: Ventricular rate determines eventual cardiac output; rapid ventricular rate may decrease cardiac output.

Treatment: Digitalization if the arrhythmia is not the result of digitalis toxicity (digitalis increases the AV block and slows the ventricular rate). Propranolol may be added. Electric cardioversion may be required. Digitalis should be discontinued for at least 48 hours before cardioversion. Quinidine may prevent recurrence.

Atrial Fibrillation

Description: Characterized by an extremely fast atrial rate ("f" wave, at a rate of 350–600 beats/min) and an irregularly irregular ventricular response with normal QRS complexes (see Fig 5–2).

Causes: Same as for atrial flutter.

Significance: Rapid ventricular rate and loss of coordinated contraction of the atria and ventricles decrease cardiac output.

Treatment: Digoxin to slow the ventricular rate. Propranolol may be added if necessary. Cardioversion may be indicated, but recurrence is common. Quinidine is used to prevent recurrence.

C. Rhythms Originating in AV Node

Rhythms originating in the AV node (Fig 5–3) show the following characteristics:

a. P wave may be absent, or inverted P waves may follow the QRS complex.
b. QRS complex is usually normal in duration and configuration.

Nodal Premature Beats

Description: P waves are usually absent, but inverted P waves may follow QRS complexes. The compensatory pause may be complete or incomplete.

Causes: Usually idiopathic in an otherwise normal heart, following cardiac surgery, and digitalis toxicity.

Significance: Usually no hemodynamic significance.

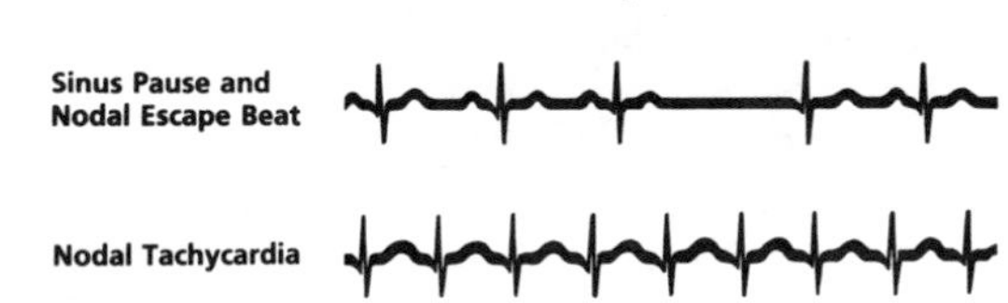

FIG 5–3.

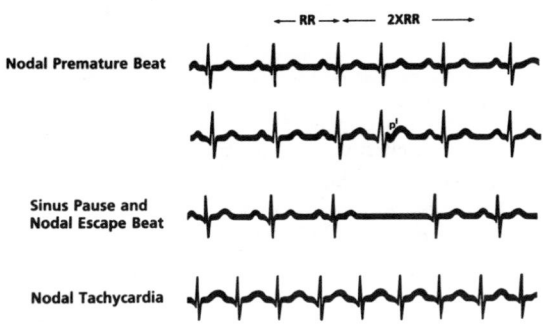

Arrhythmias originating in the AV node. (From Park MK, Guntheroth WG: *How to Read Pediatric ECGs,* ed 2. Chicago, Year Book Medical Publishers, 1987.)

Treatment: Not indicated unless caused by digitalis toxicity.

Nodal Escape Beat

Description: When the sinus node impulse fails to reach the AV node the NH region of the AV node will initiate an impulse (nodal or junctional escape beat). The QRS complex occurs later than the anticipated normal beat (see Fig 5–3).

Causes: Cardiac surgery involving the atria (Mustard or Senning procedure); may be seen in otherwise healthy children.

Significance: Little hemodynamic significance.

Treatment: Generally no specific treatment required.

Nodal or Junctional Rhythm

Description: If there is persistent failure of the sinus node, the AV node may function as the main pacemaker of the heart, with a relatively slow rate (40–60 beats/min).

Causes: Otherwise normal heart, following cardiac surgery, increased vagal tone (increased intracranial pressure, pharyngeal stimulation), and digitalis toxicity.

Significance: Slow heart rate may significantly decrease cardiac output and produce symptoms.

Treatment: Treat known causes such as digitalis toxicity. No treatment indicated if asymptomatic. Atropine or electric pacing if symptomatic.

Accelerated Nodal Rhythm

Description: In the presence of normal sinus rate and AV conduction, if the AV node (NH region) with enhanced automaticity captures the pacemaker function at a faster rate (60–120 beats/min) the rhythm is called accelerated nodal (or AV junctional) rhythm.

Causes: Idiopathic, digitalis toxicity, myocarditis, following cardiac surgery.

Significance: Little hemodynamic significance.

Treatment: No treatment necessary unless caused by digitalis toxicity.

Nodal Tachycardia

Description: Ventricular rate varies from 120 to 200 beats/min. The QRS complex is usually normal, but aberration may rarely occur. Nodal tachycardia is difficult to differentiate from atrial tachycardia; therefore both arrhythmias are grouped as supraventricular tachycardia (SVT).

Causes: Similar to those of atrial tachycardia.

Significance: May decrease cardiac output.

Treatment: Treatment not indicated if the rate is slower than 130 beats/min. Although digoxin is the drug of choice for most SVT (of atrial origin), it may be contraindicated in the true form of nodal tachycardia. In that instance, quinidine is probably the drug of choice.

D. Rhythms Originating in Ventricle

Ventricular arrhythmias are characterized by the following (Fig 5–4):

a. Bizarre, wide QRS complexes, with T waves pointing in the opposite directions.

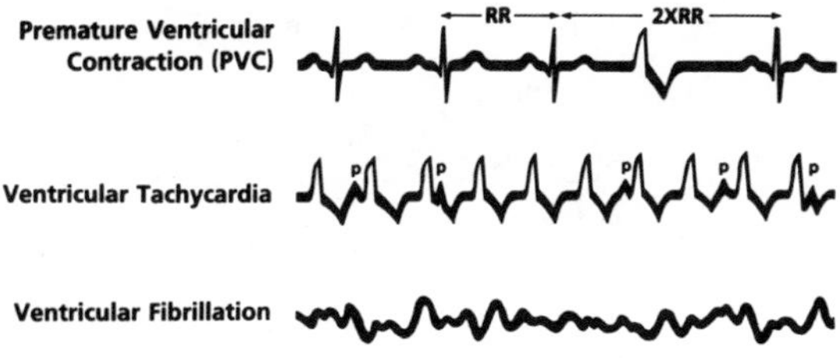

FIG 5–4.
Ventricular arrhythmias. (From Park MK, Guntheroth WG: *How to Read Pediatric ECGs,* ed 2. Chicago, Year Book Medical Publishers, 1987.)

b. QRS complexes randomly related to P waves, if visible.

Premature Ventricular Contraction (PVC)

Description: A bizarre, wide QRS complex comes earlier than anticipated, with T waves pointing in the opposite direction. There is a full compensatory pause (the length of two cycles, including the premature beat, is the same as that of two normal cycles; see Fig 5–4).

PVCs may be classified into several types, depending on the configuration, number, and regularity: (a) uniform vs. multifocal PVCs, and (b) ventricular bigeminy, trigeminy, or quadrigeminy.

Causes: Seen in otherwise healthy children; myocarditis, long QT syndrome, CHD, following heart surgery, digitalis toxicity, or drugs such as catecholamines, theophylline, caffeine, and amphetamines.

Significance: Occasional PVCs are benign in children, particularly if they are unifocal and disappear or decrease in frequency with exercise. PVCs are more likely significant if they are (1) multifocal, (2) precipitated by or increase in frequency with activity, (3) associated with underlying cardiac conditions, and (4) runs of PVCs with symptoms.

Treatment:

a. Frequent PVCs may require treatment with IV bolus injection of lidocaine (1 mg/kg/dose) followed by IV drip of lidocaine, 20–50 μg/kg/min.
b. Antiarrhythmic drugs such as propranolol, quinidine, phenytoin (Dilantin), or procainamide (Pronestyl) may be indicated.
c. PVCs that are more likely to be significant warrant electrophysiologic studies.

Ventricular Tachycardia (VT)

Description: VT is a series (six or more) of PVCs with a heart rate of 120–200 beats/min. It is sometimes difficult to differentiate VT from SVT with aberrant conduction (see below).

Causes: Similar to those listed for PVCs, except for normal children.

Significance: Usually signifies serious myocardial disease or dysfunction. Cardiac output may decrease notably, and may deteriorate to ventricular fibrillation.

Treatment:

a. Prompt synchronized cardioversion if the patient is unconscious.
b. If the patient is conscious, an IV bolus of lidocaine, 1 mg/kg/dose over 1–2 min, followed by IV drip of lidocaine, 20–50 μg/kg/min or 1–3 mg/kg/hr, may be effective.
c. Recurrence may be prevented with administration of propranolol, quinidine, or phenytoin.

Aberration

The following features are helpful in differentiating SVT with aberration from VT:

1. An rsR′ pattern in V1 and a qRs pattern in V6, resembling QRS complexes of RBBB, suggest aberration. In VT the QRS morphology is bizarre and does not resemble the classic form of RBBB or LBBB.
2. Occasional wide QRS complexes following P waves with regular PR intervals suggest an aberration.
3. The presence of ventricular "*fusion*" complex is a reliable sign of ventricular ectopic rhythm. This is a QRS complex that is produced in part by a normally conducted supraventricular impulse and in part by an ectopic ventricular impulse. The resulting QRS complex is intermediate in appearance between the patient's normal conducted beat and the pure ectopic ventricular beat.

Ventricular Fibrillation

Description: Ventricular fibrillation is characterized by bizarre QRS complexes of varying size and configuration. The rate is rapid and irregular.

Causes: Postoperative, severe hypoxia, hyperkalemia, digitalis or quinidine toxicity, myocarditis, myocardial infarction, and drugs (e.g., catecholamines, anesthetics).

Significance: Usually the terminal arrhythmia, since it results in ineffective circulation.

Treatment: Immediate CPR procedures, including electric defibrillation at the dose of 2 w·sec/kg.

II. DISTURBANCES OF ATRIOVENTRICULAR CONDUCTION

Atrioventricular block (AV block) is classified into three classes depending on the severity of the conduction disturbance: first degree, second degree, and third degree (Fig 5–5).

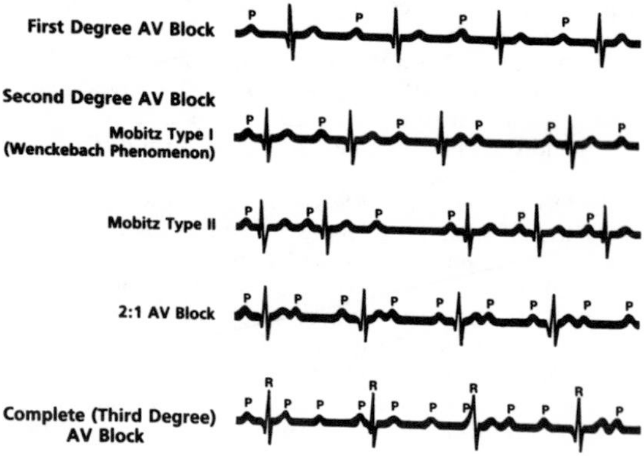

FIG 5–5.

Atrioventricular block. (From Park MK, Guntheroth WG: *How to Read Pediatric ECGs*, ed 2. Chicago, Year Book Medical Publishers, 1987.)

First-degree AV Block

Description: There is prolongation of the PR interval beyond the upper limits of normal due to an abnormal delay in conduction through the AV node (see Fig 5–5).

Causes: Acute rheumatic fever, cardiomyopathies, CHD (e.g., ASD, Ebstein's anomaly, ECD), following cardiac surgery, and digitalis toxicity; noted in some healthy children.

Significance: No hemodynamic disturbance. May progress to more advanced AV block.

Treatment: No treatment indicated unless caused by digitalis toxicity.

Second-degree AV Block

Some, but not all, P waves are followed by QRS complexes (dropped beats). There are several types:

1. *Mobitz type I (Wenckebach Phenomenon):*

   Description: The PR interval becomes progressively prolonged until one QRS complex is dropped completely (see Fig 5–5).

   Causes: Myocarditis, cardiomyopathy, MI, CHD, following surgery, and digitalis toxicity; seen in some otherwise healthy children.

   Significance: The block is at the level of the AV node. It usually does not progress to complete heart block.

   Treatment: Treat underlying causes.

2. *Mobitz type II:*

   Description: The AV conduction is "all or none": there is either normal AV conduction or the conduction is completely blocked (see Fig 5–5).

   Causes: Same as for Mobitz Type I.

   Significance: The block is at the level of His bundle. It is more serious than type I block, since it may progress to complete heart block.

   Treatment: Treat underlying causes. Prophylactic pacemaker therapy may be indicated.

3. Two-to-one (or higher) AV block:

   Description: A QRS complex follows every second (third or fourth) P wave resulting in 2:1 (3:1 or 4:1) AV block (see Fig 5–5).

Causes: Similar to other second-degree AV blocks.

Significance: The block is usually at the AV nodal level and occasionally at the level of His bundle. It may occasionally progress to complete heart block.

Treatment: Treat underlying causes. Electrophysiologic studies may be necessary to determine the level of the block. Occasional pacemaker therapy.

Third-degree AV Block (complete heart block)

Description: In third-degree AV block the atrial and ventricular activities are entirely independent of each other (see Fig 5–5): The P waves are regular (regular PP interval) with a rate comparable to the heart rate for the patient's age. The QRS complexes are also quite regular (regular RR interval) with a rate much slower than the P rate.

In congenital complete heart block the duration of the QRS complex is normal (since the pacemaker for the QRS complex is at a level higher than the bifurcation of the His bundle). The ventricular rate is faster (50–80 beats/min) than in the acquired type. In surgically induced or acquired (post-MI) complete heart block the QRS duration is prolonged and the ventricular rate is in the range of 40–50 beats/min. The pacemaker for the QRS complex is at the level below the bifurcation of the His bundle.

Causes:

a. Congenital type: An isolated anomaly (without associated CHD), maternal lupus erythematosus or mixed connective tissue disease, or CHD such as L-TGA.
b. Acquired type: As a complication of cardiac surgery in children. Rarely severe myocarditis, acute rheumatic fever, mumps, diphtheria, cardiomyopathies, tumors in the conduction system, overdose of certain drugs, and following

MI. Some of these causes may produce temporary heart block.

Significance: CHF may develop in infancy, particularly when there is associated CHD. Patients with isolated congenital heart block are usually asymptomatic during childhood. Syncopal attacks (Stokes-Adams attack) or sudden death may occur with the heart rate below 40–45 beats/min.

Treatment:

a. No treatment is required for asymptomatic children with congenital complete heart block. Atropine or isoproterenol in symptomatic children and adults until temporary ventricular pacing is secured.
b. A temporary transvenous ventricular pacemaker is indicated in patients with heart block or prophylactically in those patients who might develop heart block. A permanent artificial ventricular pacemaker is indicated in patients with surgically induced heart block and in patients with congenital heart block who are symptomatic or have CHF.

CARDIAC PROBLEMS IN THE NEWBORN

VI

The majority of cardiology consultations are requested during the newborn period for one or more of the following reasons: (a) abnormal cardiovascular findings, including heart murmur, (b) cyanosis, (c) abnormal CXRs, (d) abnormal ECGs, (e) possible CHF, and (f) cardiac arrhythmias.

I. ABNORMAL CARDIOVASCULAR FINDINGS AND HEART MURMURS

The following abnormal physical findings suggest the presence of cardiovascular malformations:

1. A heart murmur may be a presenting sign of CHD, but it could be an innocent murmur (see the following discussion).
2. Tachypnea with respiratory rate greater than 60/min with or without retraction.
3. Cyanosis, particularly when it does not improve with oxygen administration.
4. Peripheral pulses: Decreased or absent peripheral pulses in the lower extremities suggest COA. Generalized weak peripheral pulses suggest HLHS or circulatory shock. Bounding peripheral pulses suggest PDA or persistent truncus arteriosus.
5. Hepatomegaly may suggest CHF. A midline liver suggests asplenia or polysplenia syndrome.
6. Irregular rhythm and abnormal heart rate.

A. Innocent Heart Murmur

More than 50% of full-term newborn infants (and a higher percentage of premature infants) have an innocent systolic murmur at some time during the first week of life. Infants with innocent heart murmurs have normal ECG and CXR. The four most common innocent murmurs in the newborn period are as follows:

1. **Pulmonary flow murmur of the newborn** is the most common innocent heart murmur in the newborn infant. It is more common in premature and small-for-gestational-age infants than in full-term infants. A soft systolic murmur (grade 1–2/6) is heard best at the ULSB and transmits well to both sides of the chest, axillae, and the back.
2. **Transient systolic murmur of PDA** is a soft systolic murmur (grade 1–2/6) audible at the ULSB and in the left infraclavicular area on the first day. It usually disappears shortly thereafter.
3. **Transient systolic murmur of tricuspid regurgitation** is indistinguishable from that of VSD and is more common in infants who had fetal distress or neonatal asphyxia.
4. **Vibratory systolic innocent murmur** is a counterpart of Still's murmur in older children.

B. Pathologic Heart Murmur

Most pathologic murmurs should be audible during the first month of life, with the exception of ASD. Differences in the time of appearance of a heart murmur depend on the nature of the defect.

1. Heart murmurs due to stenotic lesions (e.g., AS, PS) are audible immediately after birth and persist.
2. Heart murmurs due to L–R shunt lesions, especially a large VSD, may appear later, when the PVR decreases. The murmur of ASD appears late in infancy or childhood.
3. The continuous murmur of a large PDA may not appear for 2–3 weeks. Instead, it is a crescendo systolic murmur with slight or no diastolic component.

Even in the absence of a heart murmur, a newborn infant may have a serious heart defect that requires immediate attention (e.g., severe cyanotic heart disease, such as TGA or pulmonary atresia with a closing PDA). In infants with severe CHF the murmur may not be loud until the myocardial function is improved with anticongestive measures.

II. CYANOSIS IN THE NEWBORN

Detection: Most patients with severe forms of CHD have cyanosis at birth. Early detection of cyanosis in a newborn is crucial. When in doubt, blood gases for Po_2 or transcutaneous oxygen saturation should be obtained to confirm or rule out central cyanosis. Normal 1-day-old infants may have a Po_2 as low as 60 mm Hg, but O_2 saturation is higher than 90%.

Etiology: Central cyanosis (with low arterial Po_2) may be due to (a) CNS depression, (b) lung disease, or (c) cyanotic CHD. Table 6–1 lists some of the causes and characteristic physical and laboratory findings for each type of cyanosis.

Suggested Approach in Neonates With Central Cyanosis:

1. Chest x-ray films: CXRs may reveal pulmonary causes of cyanosis and urgency of the problem. It will also hint at the presence or absence of and the type of cardiac defects.
2. Arterial blood gases in room air: These will confirm or rule out central cyanosis. Elevated Pco_2 suggests pulmonary or CNS problems. Low pH may be seen in sepsis, circulatory shock, or severe hypoxemia.
3. Hyperoxitest: Repeating arterial blood gases while breathing 100% oxygen helps to differentiate cardiac causes of cyanosis from pulmonary or CNS causes. With pulmonary or CNS diseases, arterial Po_2 usually rises to more than 100 mm Hg. When there is significant intracardiac R–L shunt, the arterial Po_2 does not exceed 100 mm Hg, and the

TABLE 6–1.

Causes and Clinical Characteristics of Central Cyanosis

A. CNS depression:
   Causes: Perinatal asphyxia, heavy maternal sedation, intrauterine fetal distress, etc.
   Findings: Shallow irregular respiration, poor muscle tone. Cyanosis disappears when the infant is stimulated or given oxygen.

B. Pulmonary disease:
   Causes: Parenchymal lung disease (e.g., hyaline membrane disease, atelectasis), pneumothorax or pleural effusion, diaphragmatic hernia, and PPHN (or PFC syndrome).
   Findings: Tachypnea and respiratory distress with retraction and expiratory grunting, rales or decreased breath sounds on auscultation; CXRs may reveal causes (as listed above). Oxygen administration improves or abolishes cyanosis.

C. Cardiac disease:
   Causes: Cyanotic CHD with R–L shunt.
   Findings: Tachypnea, but usually without retraction. No rales or abnormal breath sounds unless CHF supervenes.
   Heart murmur may be absent in serious forms of cyanotic CHD.
   A continuous murmur (of PDA) may indicate restricted PBF through the ductus.
   CXRs may show cardiomegaly, abnormal cardiac silhouette, increased or decreased PVM.
   Little or no increase in Po_2 with oxygen administration.

rise is not more than 10–30 mm Hg with cyanotic CHD.

4. ECG if cardiac origin of cyanosis is suspected.
5. Umbilical artery line: Po_2 value in a preductal artery (such as right radial artery) higher than that in a postductal artery (umbilical artery line) by 10–15 mm Hg suggests an R–L shunt through a PDA.
6. Prostaglandin E_1: If cyanotic CHD is suspected based on the above laboratory tests, alprostadil (Prostin VR Pediatric; PGE_1) should be started or made available. The starting dose is 0.05–0.1 μg/kg/min, administered by continuous IV drip.

When the desired effects (increased Po_2, increased systemic blood pressure, improved pH) are achieved, the dose should be reduced step-by-step to 0.01 μg/kg/min. When there is no effect with the initial starting dose, it may be increased to 0.4 μg/kg/min. Three common side effects of IV infusion of alprostadil are apnea (12%), fever (14%), and flushing (10%).

7. Cardiology consultation if cardiac origin of cyanosis is suspected.

Discussion of individual cyanotic heart defect is found in Chapter 3. Only persistent pulmonary hypertension of the newborn (PPHN) is discussed here.

Persistent Pulmonary Hypertension of the Newborn (PPHN; persistence of fetal circulation, PFC syndrome)

Etiology: Causes of PPHN are listed in Table 6–2.

Pathophysiology: This neonatal condition is characterized by cyanosis in the absence of intracardiac defects. An R–L shunt occurs through the PDA or the PFO, with persistence of pulmonary hypertension.

Clinical Manifestations:

1. The idiopathic form usually affects full-term or postterm neonates. There is usually a history of meconium staining or birth asphyxia.
2. Cyanosis and tachypnea (with grunting and retraction) are always present. The S2 is loud and single with increased RV impulse. A faint systolic murmur of TR, systemic hypotension, or even CHF may be present.
3. Arterial Po_2 is lower in the descending aorta or legs than in the right arm (because of R–L ductal shunt), and differential cyanosis may be evident (pink upper body and cyanotic lower part of the body). No difference in Po_2 at the two sites may be the result of an R–L shunt predominantly at the atrial level.
4. ECG is usually normal for age, but occasional

TABLE 6–2.

Causes of Persistent Pulmonary Hypertension of the Newborn

1. Pulmonary vasoconstriction in the presence of a normally developed pulmonary vascular bed may be caused by or seen in:
   a. Alveolar hypoxia (meconium aspiration syndrome, hyaline membrane disease, hypoventilation due to CNS anomalies)
   b. Birth asphyxia
   c. LV dysfunction or circulatory shock
   d. Infections (such as group B hemolytic streptococcal infection)
   e. Hyperviscosity syndrome (polycythemia)
   f. Hypoglycemia and hypocalcemia
2. Increased pulmonary vascular smooth muscle development (hypertrophy) may be caused by:
   a. Chronic intrauterine asphyxia
   b. Maternal use of PG synthesis inhibitors (aspirin, indomethacin) results in early ductal closure
3. Decreased cross-sectional area of pulmonary vascular bed may be seen in association with:
   a. Congenital diaphragmatic hernia
   b. Primary pulmonary hypoplasia

RVH or T wave changes suggestive of myocardial dysfunction may be present.

5. CXRs reveal varying degrees of cardiomegaly, with or without findings suggestive of meconium aspiration.
6. Echo studies show no evidence of cyanotic CHD but the presence of a large PDA. An R–L shunt is detected by Doppler studies at the ductal or atrial level (PFO or ASD). CHD such as preductal COA or interrupted aortic arch should be ruled out.

Treatment: The goal of therapy is to lower PVR by administration of oxygen and induction of respiratory alkalosis by the use of a respirator, and by administration of pulmonary vasodilators (such as tolazoline). Dopamine or dobutamine is often used to improve cardiac function. Correction of hypocalcemia, hypoglycemia, and acidosis is important. Extracorporeal membrane oxygenation (ECMO) is effective in selected patients with severe PPHN.

III. ABNORMAL CHEST X-RAY FILMS

Abnormal CXRs suggestive of CHD may include abnormalities of the cardiac shadow itself, abdominal viscera, or pulmonary vascularity.

A. Abnormal Heart Size, Silhouette, and Position:

1. Unequivocal cardiomegaly may be due to CHD, myocarditis or cardiomyopathy, pericardial effusion, severe hypoxemia and acidosis, and overhydration or overtransfusion.
2. Abnormal cardiac silhouette:
   a. "Boot-shaped" heart (with decreased PVM) is seen in TOF or tricuspid atresia.
   b. "Egg-shaped" heart with narrow waist (and increased PVM) may be seen in TGA.
   c. A large globular heart is seen with Ebstein's anomaly.
3. Dextrocardia or mesocardia. Four common situations in which the heart is located in the right side of the chest or in the midline are as follows (see Fig 3–8, and chapter 3 for further discussion):
   a. Situs inversus totalis with normal heart.
   b. Hypoplasia of the right lung with displacement toward the right of a normally formed heart.
   c. Complex cyanotic heart defect, including atrial or ventricular inversion.
   d. Asplenia or polysplenia syndrome with midline liver.

B. Abnormalities of Abdominal Viscera:

1. A midline liver indicates asplenia or polysplenia syndrome with complex cyanotic CHD.
2. A left-sided liver with the heart in the right side of

the chest may indicate situs inversus totalis with mirror-image dextrocardia.
3. The liver and the cardiac apex on the same side usually suggest complex cardiac defects.

C. Abnormal Pulmonary Vascular Markings:

1. Increased PVMs in a cyanotic infant suggest TGA, persistent truncus arteriosus, or single ventricle. In an acyanotic newborn infant increased PVMs suggest VSD, PDA, or ECD.
2. Decreased PVMs with "black" lung fields suggest critical cyanotic CHD, such as pulmonary atresia, tricuspid atresia, or TOF with pulmonary atresia. Decreased PVMs with marked cardiomegaly are seen in Ebstein's anomaly.
3. "Ground glass" appearance or a reticulated pattern of lung fields is characteristic of pulmonary venous obstruction and suggests HLHS or TAPVR with obstruction.

IV. ABNORMAL ECGS

Any of the following ECG abnormalities may suggest CHD, although normal neonates may occasionally exhibit some of these abnormalities. Normal ECGs by no means rule out CHD.

A. Abnormal P and QRS Axes:

1. Abnormal P axis:
   a. A P axis in the right lower quadrant (+90 to +180 degrees) suggests atrial situs inversus, asplenia syndrome, or incorrectly placed electrodes.
   b. A "superior" P axis (negative P in aVF) suggests ectopic atrial rhythm or polysplenia syndrome.
2. Abnormal QRS axis:
   a. "Superior" QRS axis suggests ECD, tricuspid atresia, or splenic syndromes (asplenia or polysplenia).

b. Definite LAD ($<+30$ degrees) or relative LAD (between $+30$ and $+60$ degrees) in a neonate may occur with LVH.
c. QRS axis greater than $+180$ degrees (in the range of -150 degrees to -180 degrees) may indicate RAD. It may occur with RVH or RBBB.

B. Ventricular and Atrial Hypertrophy:

1. LVH is suggested when the following are present:
   a. LAD or relative LAD ($<+60$ degrees).
   b. R/S progression in precordial leads that resembles the adult R/S progression.
   c. QRS voltages demonstrating abnormal leftward and posterior forces or abnormal inferior forces for age.
2. RVH is difficult to diagnose because of the normal dominance of the RV at this age. However, the following are helpful clues to RVH in the newborn.
   a. Pure R wave (with no S wave) in V1 >10 mm.
   b. R in V1 >25 mm or R in aVR >8 mm.
   c. qR pattern in V1 (also present in 10% of normal newborns).
   d. Upright T in V1 after 3 days of age.
   e. RAD greater than $+180$ degrees.
3. Atrial hypertrophy:
   a. RAH is present when P wave amplitude is greater than 3 mm in any lead.
   b. LAH is present when P wave duration is 0.08 seconds or greater (usually with notched P waves in the limb leads and biphasic P waves in V1).

C. Ventricular Conduction Disturbance:

Ventricular conduction disturbance (such as RBBB, LBBB, WPW syndrome) is present when the QRS duration is greater than 0.07 seconds.

1. RBBB may be seen in Ebstein's anomaly, COA in infants, ASD, PAPVR, or normal neonates.

2. LBBB is extremely rare in the newborn.
3. Intraventricular block (wide QRS complex throughout the QRS duration) is often associated with metabolic abnormalities (hypoxia, acidosis, hyperkalemia), diffuse myocardial disease, occasionally with CHD, or as a terminal ECG in a dying patient.
4. WPW syndrome may be an isolated finding or may be associated with CHD (Ebstein's anomaly or L-TGA), and is a frequent cause of SVT.

V. HEART FAILURE IN THE NEWBORN

The clinical picture of CHF in the newborn period may simulate other disorders, such as meningitis, sepsis, pneumonia, or bronchiolitis. Tachypnea, tachycardia, pulmonary rales or rhonchi, hepatomegaly, and weak peripheral pulses are common presenting signs. Heart murmur is frequently absent. Cardiomegaly, with or without increased PVMs or pulmonary edema on CXR is always present. Causes of CHF in the newborn are listed in Table 6–3. The time of onset of CHF varies rather predictably with the type of CHD. Detailed discussion of treatment of CHF is presented in chapter 7.

Two important structural abnormalities of the cardiovascular system that are seen with CHF in the newborn period are hypoplastic left heart syndrome (HLHS) and large PDA in premature infants.

A. Hypoplastic Left Heart Syndrome (HLHS)

Incidence: One percent to 2% of all CHD. The most common cause of death from CHD during the first month of life.

Pathology and Pathophysiology:

1. This syndrome includes a group of closely related anomalies characterized by hypoplasia of the LV (from atresia or severe stenosis of the aortic and/or mitral valve) and hypoplasia of the aortic arch.
2. During fetal life the PVR is higher than the SVR and the dominant RV maintains normal perfusing

TABLE 6–3.

Causes of Heart Failure in the Newborn

A. Structural heart defects
   At birth
      Hypoplastic left heart syndrome (HLHS)
      Severe tricuspid or pulmonary regurgitation
      Large systemic AV fistula
   Week 1
      TGA
      Large PDA in premature infant
      TAPVR below diaphragm
   Weeks 1–4
      Critical AS or PS
      Preductal COA
B. Noncardiac causes
   1. Birth asphyxia (resulting in transient myocardial ischemia)
   2. Metabolic: hypoglycemia, hypocalcemia
   3. Severe anemia (as seen in hydrops fetalis)
   4. Neonatal sepsis
   5. Overtransfusion or overhydration
C. Primary myocardial disease
   1. Myocarditis
   2. Transient myocardial ischemia (with or without birth asphyxia)
   3. Cardiomyopathy (seen in infants of diabetic mothers)
D. Disturbances in heart rate
   1. Supraventricular tachycardia (SVT or PAT)
   2. Atrial flutter or fibrillation
   3. Congenital heart block (when associated with CHD)

pressure in the descending aorta through the ductal R–L shunt, even in the presence of the nonfunctioning hypoplastic LV. However, difficulties arise after birth, primarily from two factors: (a) reversal of the vascular resistance in the two circuits, with higher SVR than the PVR, and (b) closure of the PDA. The end result is a marked decrease in systemic cardiac output and aortic pressure producing circulatory shock and metabolic acidosis. An increase in PBF in the presence of the nonfunctioning LV results in an elevated LA pressure and pulmonary edema.

Clinical Manifestations:

1. Critically ill in the first few hours to days of life, with mild cyanosis, tachycardia, tachypnea, and pulmonary rales.
2. Poor peripheral pulses and vasoconstricted extremities are characteristic. The S2 is loud and single. Heart murmur is usually absent, but a grade 1–3/6 nonspecific systolic murmur may be present over the precordium.
3. ECG shows RVH.
4. CXRs show pulmonary venous congestion or pulmonary edema. The heart is only mildly enlarged.
5. Arterial blood gas determination reveals severe metabolic acidosis in the presence of slightly decreased Po_2, a characteristic finding of this condition.
6. Echo findings are diagnostic and usually obviate cardiac catheterization. Severe hypoplasia of the aorta and aortic annulus and absent or distorted mitral valve are usually imaged. The LV cavity is diminutive. The RV cavity is markedly dilated and the tricuspid valve is large.
7. Progressive hypoxemia and acidosis, resulting in death, usually in the first month of life.

Management:

Medical:

a. Intubation, adminstration of oxygen, and correction of metabolic acidosis.
b. IV infusion of PGE_1 (Prostin VR Pediatric) may produce temporary improvement by reopening the ductus arteriosus.

Surgical: Surgical procedures still carry high mortality.

a. The first-stage Norwood operation (mortality >75%; Fig 6–1) is followed by a Fontan-type operation at 6–24 months of age (mortality up to 50%). The Fontan-type operation involves (a) closure of the Gore-Tex shunt, (b) direct

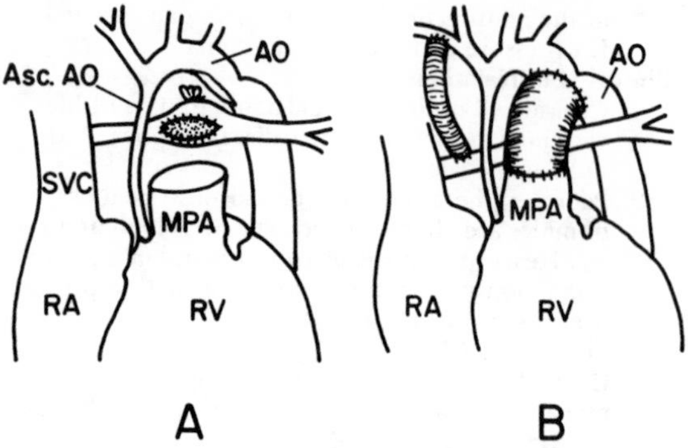

FIG 6–1.
Norwood operation. **A,** MPA is divided, and the distal PA is closed. **B,** proximal MPA is connected to the descending aorta with the use of conduit. A right-sided Gore-Tex shunt procedure is performed. A large ASD is created by surgery at the same time. (From Park MK: *Pediatric Cardiology for Practitioners,* ed 2. Chicago, Year Book Medical Publishers, 1988.)

anastomosis between the RA or SVC and the PA, and (c) closure of the surgically created ASD.

b. Cardiac transplantation is experimental.

B. Heart Failure in Premature Infants With PDA

Pathophysiology: This represents a special problem in premature infants who have been recovering from hyaline membrane disease. With improvement in oxygenation, the PVR drops rapidly, but the ductus remains patent. The resulting large L–R ductal shunt makes the lungs stiff, and the infant becomes respirator-dependent. Infants who remain on the respirator and oxygen therapy for an extended period of time develop bronchopulmonary dysplasia with resulting pulmonary hypertension (cor pulmonale) and right heart failure.

Clinical Manifestations:

1. History usually reveals that a premature infant with hyaline membrane disease has made some improvement during the first few days after birth, but this is followed by inability to wean the infant from the respirator or a need to increase ventilator settings or oxygen requirement in 4- to 7-day-old premature infants. Apneic spells or episodes of bradycardia may be initial signs in infants who are not on a ventilator.
2. Bounding peripheral pulses and hyperactive precordium are usually present. The classic continuous murmur of PDA at the ULSB is diagnostic, but the murmur is sometimes systolic only at the middle and upper LSB.
3. ECG is usually normal.
4. CXRs show cardiomegaly and evidence of pulmonary edema or pulmonary venous congestion, in addition to varying degrees of the lung disease.
5. 2D Echo and Doppler study confirm the diagnosis. 2D Echo actually images the PDA, and the Doppler study (and color flow mapping) confirms the presence of an L–R ductal shunt. Indirect estimate of the magnitude of the shunt can be made by measuring LA and LV dimensions by M-mode or 2D Echo.

Management: For symptomatic infants, either pharmacologic (indomethacin) or surgical closure of the ductus is indicated. A small PDA that is not causing CHF should be followed up medically for 6 months without surgical ligation because of the possibility of spontaneous closure of PDA.

VI. ARRHYTHMIAS OF THE NEWBORN

Although once thought to be rare, arrhythmias are not uncommon in healthy premature and full-term newborn infants.

Sinus arrhythmia is common in healthy full-term and premature infants. It has no clinical significance.

Sinus tachycardia: Transient tachycardia with rates up to 180–190 beats/min is commonly seen in normal newborns and does not require treatment. Persistent tachycardia may be caused by hypovolemia, hyperthermia, catecholamines, theophylline, or hyperthyroidism. Detection and correction of the underlying cause is indicated.

Sinus bradycardia: Transient bradycardia (<70 beats/min) may be seen in normal neonates and requires no treatment. Prolonged bradycardia may be related to apnea (either preceded or followed by), maternal medications (e.g., reserpine), or neonatal asphyxia. Treatment should be directed to correct or improve underlying cause.

Sinus pause or arrest may occasionally occur in normal full-term and premature neonates, but digitalis toxicity or hyperkalemia should be considered a possibility.

Wandering atrial pacemaker may occur in healthy newborn infants and does not require therapy.

Premature contractions are common, occurring in as many as 30% of healthy premature and full-term neonates. Supraventricular (atrial or nodal) premature contractions are encountered more frequently than PVCs. These premature contractions are occasionally associated with CHDs, severe respiratory distress syndrome, sepsis, digitalis toxicity, or hypoxemia.

Treatment is not indicated unless they are frequent PVCs. Treatment should be directed to correcting the underlying causes, such as digitalis toxicity, sepsis, or hypoxemia. Frequent PVCs may be treated with intravenous lidocaine or oral phenytoin (Dilantin).

Supraventricular tachycardia (SVT) is the most frequently encountered arrhythmia of significance in the newborn period. The heart rate is usually 240 ± 40 beats/min, with a normal-appearing QRS complex. WPW syndrome is responsible in about 50% of neonatal cases. Structural heart diseases (such as Ebstein's anomaly, tricuspid atresia, and cardiac tumors), viral myocarditis, and thyrotoxicosis are less frequent causes of SVT in neonates.

Newborns with SVT usually develop signs of CHF within 24–48 hours after onset. They are restless and tachypneic or "wheezy," and eventually develop signs of CHF (pallor, apathy, circulatory shock).

Cardioversion is the treatment of choice when CHF is present in a neonate, followed by digitalization and diuretics. Transesophageal electric stimulation may prove as safe and equally effective as cardioversion. In SVT of short duration without signs of CHF, digoxin alone is used. Application of an icebag on the face has been used successfully in the neonate. Verapamil or propranolol is not the drug of choice and is indicated only when other measures fail. They should be given step-by-step in a small dose with careful monitoring and readiness to resuscitate the infant.

Atrial flutter or fibrillation is a relatively rare arrhythmia, often associated with CHD (such as Ebstein's anomaly, MS, tricuspid atresia), viral myocarditis, and systemic infections. Severe CHF may develop. Cardioversion is the treatment of choice in infants who are in CHF, followed by digoxin. In the infant without CHF, the use of digoxin is indicated to prevent CHF by controlling the ventricular rate within an acceptable range.

Ventricular tachycardia is rare but more serious than any other arrhythmia. It may be associated with CHD, myocarditis, cardiomyopathy, or cardiac tumors, as well as hyperkalemia or asphyxia. Treatment consists of termination of the arrhythmia with lidocaine infusion or cardioversion, correction of the underlying cause when possible, and prevention of recurrence with antiarrhythmic agents (phenytoin, propranolol).

Atrioventricular block

1. First-degree AV block (prolongation of PR interval) may be benign, although it may be a sign of digitalis toxicity, CHD (ECD, ASD, Ebstein's anomaly), or metabolic abnormalities.
2. Second-degree AV block is a sign of digitalis toxicity until proved otherwise.

3. Third-degree AV block (complete heart block) is due to a structural defect in the conduction system, usually above the bifurcation of the His bundle (with narrow QRS complexes). About one third of cases are associated with CHD. There is frequent association of maternal lupus erythematosus or mixed connective tissue disease, with congenital complete heart block in the offspring. When associated with CHD, resulting in CHF, pacemaker therapy is required. When not associated with CHD, treatment is usually not indicated until childhood.

SPECIAL PROBLEMS

VII

I. CHEST PAIN

In office or emergency room practice, chest pain is a frequently encountered complaint in children. Although in the majority of pediatric patients chest pain does not indicate serious disease of the heart or other systems, chest pain means "heart disease" to the majority of these children and their parents. Making a referral to a cardiologist is not always a good idea; it may actually increase the family's concern. Physicians should be aware of the differential diagnosis of chest pain in children and should make every effort to find a specific cause of chest pain before reassuring the child and parents.

Etiology:

Causes of chest pain in children are listed in Table 7–1. Costochondritis is the most common cause (20%–75%), followed by trauma to the chest wall or muscle strain, and respiratory diseases associated with cough. Cardiac diseases are rarely seen with chest pain in children. No cause is found in 40% of patients even after moderately extensive studies. Psychologic cause of chest pain should not be lightly assigned to these children without thorough history taking and follow-up evaluation.

Evaluation:

1. Careful history taking and physical examination reveal causes of chest pain in the majority of patients.
2. Cardiac causes of chest pain should be ruled out (by physical examination, ECG, and CXR).
3. Cardiology consultation is occasionally indicated, if cardiac origin of chest pain is suspected. Echo and Doppler studies and exercise tolerance test may be indicated.

TABLE 7–1.

Causes of Chest Pain in Children

Cardiac
Structural heart defects
Severe obstructive lesions (severe AS, PS, HOCM)
Pulmonary vascular obstructive disease
Mitral valve prolapse(?)
Anomalous origin of the coronary artery
Inflammatory
Pericarditis (viral, bacterial, rheumatic)
Kawasaki's disease
Arrhythmias(?) (SVT, frequent PVCs or VT)
Thoracic cage
Costochondritis
Muscle strain or direct trauma to the chest wall
Breast tenderness (mastalgia)
Abnormalities of rib cage or thoracic spine
Respiratory
Severe cough or bronchitis
Pleural effusion, lobar pneumonia, spontaneous pneumothorax
Pleurodynia or other viral infection
Drug abuse (e.g., cocaine)
Psychogenic (hyperventilation, conversion symptoms, somatization disorder, depression)

II. SYNCOPE

Normal function of the brain depends on a constant supply of oxygen and glucose. Significant alterations in their supply may result in a transient loss or near-loss of consciousness, called syncope or fainting.

Etiology:

Syncope may be due to circulatory, metabolic, or neuropsychologic causes. Table 7–2 lists possible causes of syncope.

Evaluation:

If cardiac causes of syncope are suspected, complete cardiac evaluation, including ECG, CXR, and Echo and Doppler studies, is indicated. A 24-hour ambulatory

TABLE 7–2.

Etiologic Classification of Syncope

- Circulatory causes
  - Extracardiac causes
    - Common faint (or vasodepressor syncope)
    - Orthostatic hypotension
    - Failure of venous return (e.g., increased intrathoracic pressure, decreased venous return, hypovolemia)
    - Cerebrovascular occlusive disease
  - Intracardiac causes
    - Severe obstructive lesions (e.g., AS, PS, HOCM, pulmonary hypertension)
    - Arrhythmias (either extreme tachycardia or bradycardia)
- Metabolic causes
  - Hypoglycemia
  - Hyperventilation syndrome
  - Hypoxia
- Neuropsychiatric causes
  - Epilepsy
  - Brain tumor
  - Migraine
  - Hysteria or nonconvulsive seizures

ECG or an exercise tolerance test may occasionally be indicated to document causal relationship between arrhythmias and symptoms.

III. CONGESTIVE HEART FAILURE (CHF)

Etiology: CHF may result from congenital or acquired heart diseases or from myocardial insufficiency.

1. CHD as a cause of CHF is presented in Table 7–3 according to the age at which CHF usually develops.
2. Acquired heart disease: (a) acute rheumatic carditis (in school-aged children); (b) valvular rheumatic heart disease (in older children and adults).
3. Myocardial dysfunction of various causes: (a) viral myocarditis (more common in small children and

TABLE 7–3.

Causes of CHF Due to CHD According to Age

Birth:	a. HLHS b. Volume overload lesions (such as severe TR or PR, and large systemic AV fistula)
1st Week	a. TGA b. PDA in small premature infants c. HLHS (with more favorable anatomy) d. TAPVR, particularly those with pulmonary venous obstruction e. Others (systemic AV fistula, critical AS or PS)
1–4 Weeks	a. COA (preductal, with associated anomalies) b. Critical AS c. Large L–R shunt lesions (VSD, PDA) in premature infants d. All other lesions listed above
4–6 Weeks	Some L–R shunt lesions such as ECD
6 Weeks–4 Months	a. Large VSD b. Large PDA c. Others such as anomalous left coronary artery from the PA

newborns); (b) endocardial fibroelastosis (infancy); (c) anomalous left coronary artery from PA with myocardial infarction (2–3 months); (d) metabolic abnormalities (severe hypoxia, acidosis, hypoglycemia, and hypocalcemia [newborn infants]; (e) congestive cardiomyopathies and other cardiomyopathies associated with muscular dystrophy or Friedreich's ataxis (older children and adolescents).

4. Miscellaneous causes: (a) SVT (early infancy); (b) congenital heart block associated with other structural heart defects (newborn or early infancy); (c) severe anemia or sicklemia (at any age), and hydrops fetalis (newborn); (d) acute hypertension seen in acute glomerulonephritis (school-aged children);

(e) bronchopulmonary dysplasia (premature infants); and (f) acute cor pulmonale (any age).

Clinical Manifestations:

The diagnosis of CHF relies on several sources of clinical findings, including history, physical examination, and CXRs. Cardiomegaly on a CXR is almost necessary for the diagnosis of CHF.

1. History of poor feeding of recent onset, tachypnea, poor weight gain, and cold sweat on the forehead.
2. Physical findings:
   a. As compensatory responses to impaired cardiac function:
      (1) Tachycardia, gallop rhythm, weak and thready pulse, and cardiomegaly.
      (2) Signs of increased sympathetic discharges (growth failure, perspiration, cold wet skin).
   b. Signs of pulmonary venous congestion (left-sided failure), including tachypnea, dyspnea on exertion (poor feeding in small infants), orthopnea in older children, and wheezing and pulmonary rales.
   c. Signs of systemic venous congestion (right-sided failure), including hepatomegaly and puffy eyelids (distended neck veins and ankle edema are not seen in infants).
3. Cardiomegaly on CXRs (absence of cardiomegaly almost rules out CHF).
4. ECGs may be helpful in determining the type of defects (but not helpful in deciding whether CHF is present).
5. Echo may confirm the presence of chamber enlargement or impaired LV function and determine the cause of CHF.

Management:

1. General measures:
   a. "Cardiac chair" and oxygen (40%–50%) with humidity.
   b. Sedation with morphine sulfate or phenobarbital for 1–2 days occasionally indicated.

c. Salt restriction. In infants, a low-salt formula and severe fluid restriction are not indicated; use of a diuretic has replaced these measures. In older children, salt restriction (<0.5 gm/day) and avoidance of salty snacks (e.g., chips, pretzels) and table salt are recommended.
d. Daily weight measurement in hospitalized patients.
e. Elimination or correction of predisposing factors (fever, anemia, infection).
f. Treatment of underlying causes (hypertension, arrhythmias, thyrotoxicosis).

2. Drug therapy:
Digitalis is almost always used in conjunction with diuretics unless its use is contraindicated (HOCM [or IHSS], complete heart block, cardiac tamponade).
   a. Digitalis glycosides:
      (1) Total digitalizing dose (TDD) and maintenance dose of digoxin are presented in Chapter 9, "Cardiovascular Drug Dosage."
      (2) The following is a suggested step-by-step method of digitalization:
         (a) Obtain a baseline ECG (rhythm and PR interval) and serum electrolyte values.
         (b) Give one half TDD stat, followed by one fourth and the final one fourth of the TDD at 6–8 hour intervals.
         (c) Start the maintenance dose 12 hours after the final TDD.
         (d) Obtain ECGs to rule out digoxin toxicity before the final one fourth TDD or the first maintenance dose.
      (3) Monitoring for digitalis toxicity:
      Detection of digitalis toxicity is best accomplished by ECG monitoring (Table 7–4). In general, digitalis *effect* is confined to ventricular repolarization; *toxicity* involves disturbances in the formation and conduction of the impulse. A

TABLE 7–4.

ECG Changes Associated With Digitalis

Effects:
- Shortening of QTc is the earliest sign of digitalis effect.
- Sagging ST segment and diminished amplitude of T wave (T vector does not change).
- Slowing of heart rate.

Toxicity:
- Prolongation of PR interval.
  - Some normal children have prolonged PR interval, making it mandatory to obtain a baseline ECG. May progress to advanced AV block.
- Profound sinus bradycardia or sinoatrial block.
- Supraventricular arrhythmias (atrial or nodal ectopic beats and tachycardias), particularly if accompanied by AV block, are more common than ventricular arrhythmias in children.
- Ventricular arrhythmias are extremely rare in children, although common in adults with digitalis toxicity.
- PVCs are not uncommon in children as a sign of toxicity.

sound rule is to assume that any arrhythmia or conduction disturbance occurring with digitalis is caused by digitalis until proved otherwise.

Routine determination of serum digoxin levels and use of those levels for therapeutic goals are not recommended. An elevated serum level (>2 ng/ml) is likely associated with toxicity in a child if the clinical findings are suggestive of digitalis toxicity. Patients with any of the conditions listed in Table 7–5 are more likely to develop toxicity.

b. Diuretics:

Commonly used diuretics are furosemide or ethacrynic acid, and thiazide diuretics with or without aldosterone antagonist. Side effects of diuretic therapy include hypokalemia and hypochloremic alkalosis; both may increase the likelihood of digitalis toxicity (see Chapter 9, "Cardiovascular Drug Dosages").

TABLE 7–5.

Factors That May Predispose to Digitalis Toxicity

High serum digoxin level
High-dose requirement as in treatment of certain arrhythmias
Decreased renal excretion (premature infants, renal disease)
Hypothyroidism
Drug interaction (e.g., quinidine, verapamil, amiodarone)
Increased sensitivity of myocardium (without high serum digoxin level)
Status of myocardium (myocardial ischemia, rheumatic or viral myocarditis)
Systemic changes (electrolytes [↓K, ↑Ca], hypoxia, alkalosis)
Catecholamines
Immediate postoperative period after heart surgery under CPB

c. Other inotropic agents:
In infants with severe distress or those with renal dysfunction such as seen with infantile COA, rapidly acting catecholamines with short duration of action (dopamine, isoproterenol, dobutamine) are preferable to digoxin.

d. Afterload reducing agents:
These agents improve cardiac output by reducing SVR. Depending on the site of action, they may be divided into three groups: (1) venodilators (nitroglycerin, nitrates), (2) arteriolar vasodilators (hydralazine, captopril), and (3) mixed vasodilators (nitroprusside, prazosin).

3. Surgical management:
If medical treatment is not successful, specific palliative or corrective cardiac surgery should be performed.

IV. SYSTEMIC HYPERTENSION

Definition:

1. High normal BP: Average systolic or diastolic BP between the 90th and 95th percentiles for age.

2. Hypertension: Systolic or diastolic BP greater than the 95th percentile for age on at least three occasions.

World Health Organization (WHO) definition of hypertension in the adult: borderline hypertension, 140–150/90–95; hypertension, 160/95 or higher.

Etiology: Causes of hypertension are listed in Table 7–6. More than 90% of secondary hypertension in children is caused by three conditions: renal parenchymal disease, renal artery disease, and COA. In general, the younger the child and the more severe the hyperten-

TABLE 7–6.

Causes of Hypertension

A. Primary (or essential) hypertension.
B. Secondary hypertension:
   1. Renal:
      (a) Renal parenchymal disease: glomerulonephritis, pyelonephritis, polycystic or dysplastic kidneys, hydronephrosis, hemolytic uremic syndrome, collagen disease (periarteritis, lupus), renal damage from nephrotoxic medications, trauma, or radiation.
      (b) Renovascular diseases: renal artery stenosis, polyarteritis, renal artery or vein thrombosis.
   2. Cardiovascular: COA.
   3. Endocrine.
      Hyperthyroidism.
      Excessive catecholamines: pheochromocytoma, neuroblastoma.
      Adrenal dysfunction: congenital adrenal hyperplasia, Cushing's syndrome, hyperaldosteronism (primary or secondary), hyperparathyroidism.
   4. Neurogenic: increased intracranial pressure, poliomyelitis, Guillain-Barré syndrome, dysautonomia.
   5. Drugs and chemicals: sympathomimetic drugs (nose drops, cough medications, cold preparations), amphetamines, steroids, oral contraceptives, heavy metal (mercury, lead) poisoning.
   6. Miscellaneous: hypervolemia and hypernatremia, Stevens-Johnson syndrome.

sion the more likely an underlying cause can be identified.

Diagnosis and Workup:

Careful evaluation of history, physical findings, and simple laboratory tests usually point to the cause of hypertension.

1. History:
   a. Past and current history:
      (1) Neonatal: use of umbilical artery catheters.
      (2) Cardiovascular: history of COA or surgery for it. History of palpitation, headache, and excessive sweating (excessive catecholamines).
      (3) Renal: history of obstructive uropathies, urinary tract infection, radiation, trauma, or surgery to the kidney area.
      (4) Endocrine: weakness and muscle cramp (hyperaldosteronism).
      (5) Medications: corticosteroids, amphetamines, antiasthmatic drugs, cold medications, oral contraceptives, nephrotoxic antibiotics.
      (6) Habits: smoking.
   b. Family history:
      (1) Essential hypertension, atherosclerotic heart disease, cerebrovascular accident.
      (2) Familiar or hereditary renal disease (polycystic kidney, cystinuria, familial nephritis).
2. Physical examination:
   a. Accurate measurement of blood pressure is essential (See chapter 1 for method and normal BP levels).
   b. Complete physical examination, with emphasis on delayed growth (renal disease), bounding peripheral pulse (PDA or AR), weak or absent femoral pulses (COA), abdominal bruits (renovascular), and tender kidney (renal infection).
3. Laboratory tests:
   Initial laboratory tests are directed toward detecting renal parenchymal disease, renovascular disease, and COA: urinalysis, urine culture, serum electrolytes, BUN, or creatinine, uric acid, ECG, CXRs,

and possibly Echo. Children younger than 10 years of age with sustained hypertension require extensive evaluation, since identifiable and potentially curable causes are likely to be found. Adolescents with mild hypertension and positive family history of essential hypertension are more likely to have essential hypertension, and extensive studies are not indicated. Table 7–7 summarizes usefulness of the routine and more involved tests in identifying the cause of secondary hypertension.

Management:

1. Essential hypertension:
   a. Nonpharmacologic intervention initially: weight reduction, low-salt (and potassium-rich) diet, physical fitness, and avoidance of smoking and oral contraceptives.
   b. Drug therapy:
   Indications for drug therapy include family history of early complications of hypertension, the presence of target organ damage (e.g., ocular, cardiac, renal, CNS), and symptoms or signs related to elevated BP.

   The stepped-care approach is popular. Step 1 is initiated with a small dose of a single antihypertensive drug, either a diuretic (hydrochlorothiazide, chlorothiazide, furosemide, spironolactone) or an adrenergic inhibitor (e.g., propranolol, atenolol, metoprolol, methyldopa, prazosine), and then proceeds to full dose, if necessary. In black, diabetic, or asthmatic patients, the diuretic is suggested as first-step therapy. (A beta adrenergic blocker may be contraindicated in patients with diabetes or asthma; the diuretic works well in adult black patients). In adolescents with hyperdynamic-type hypertension (with rapid pulse) or in patients with associated hyperthyroidism, a beta blocker is preferable. If the first drug is not effective, a second drug may be added to or substituted for the first drug, starting with a small dose and proceeding

TABLE 7–7.

Routine and Special Laboratory Tests and Their Significance

Laboratory Test	Significance of Abnormal Results
Urinalysis, urine culture, BUN, creatinine	Renal parenchymal disease
Serum electrolytes (hypokalemia)	Hyperaldosteronism, primary or secondary
	Adrenogenital syndrome
	Renin-producing tumors
ECG, CXRs, Echo	Cardiac cause of hypertension, also baseline function
Intravenous pyelography (or ultrasonography, radionuclide studies, CT of kidneys)	Renal parenchymal disease
	Renovascular hypertension
	Tumors (neuroblastoma, Wilms' tumor)
Plasma renin activity (PRA), peripheral	High-renin hypertension
	Renovascular hypertension
	Renin-producing tumors
	Some Cushing's syndrome
	Some essential hypertension
	Low-renin hypertension
	Adrenogenital syndrome
	Primary hyperaldosteronism

24-hr urine collection for 17-KS and 17-OHCS	Cushing's syndrome
	Adrenogenital syndrome
24-Hr urine collection for catecholamines and VMA	Pheochromocytoma
	Neuroblastoma
Aldosterone	Hyperaldosteronism, primary or secondary
	Renovascular hypertension
	Renin-producing tumors
Renal vein PRA	Unilateral renal parenchymal disease
	Renovascular hypertension
Abdominal aortogram	Renovascular hypertension
	Abdominal coarctation of aorta
	Unilateral renal parenchymal diseases
	Pheochromocytoma

to full dose (step 2). If BP still remains elevated, a third drug, such as vasodilator (hydralazine, minoxidil) or captopril may be added to the regimen (step 3). Dosages of commonly used antihypertensive drugs for children are given in Chapter 9, "Cardiovascular Drug Dosage."

2. Secondary hypertension:
   Treatment of secondary hypertension should be aimed at removing the cause of hypertension whenever possible. Medical management discussed above can control hypertension caused by most renal parenchymal diseases. Concomitant antibiotic therapy for infectious processes may be indicated. Unilateral renal parenchymal disease may be treated with unilateral nephrectomy. Renovascular disease may be cured by successful surgery (reconstruction of a stenotic renal artery, autotransplantation, or unilateral nephrectomy). Hypertension caused by tumors (pheochromocytoma, neuroblastoma) is treated primarily by surgery. Surgical repair or balloon angioplasty is indicated in COA.

Hypertensive Crisis

1. In a patient with severe hypertension (>180 mm Hg systolic or >110 mm Hg diastolic), any of the following features indicates a hypertensive emergency:
   a. Neurologic signs with severe headache, vomiting, irritability, or apathy, seizures, papilledema, retinal hemorrhage, or exudate (hypertensive encephalopathy).
   b. CHF or pulmonary edema.
2. Aggressive parenteral administration of antihypertensive drugs is indicated to lower blood pressure.
   a. Diazoxide (Hyperstat), 1–3 mg/kg IV bolus, or nitroprusside (Nipride), 2–3 μg/kg/min IV drip, is the treatment of choice.
   b. If hypertension is less severe, hydralazine (Apresoline), 0.15 mg/kg IV or IM, may be used. The dose may be repeated at 4–6 hour intervals.

c. A rapid-acting diuretic, such as furosemide, 1 mg/kg IV, is given to initiate diuresis.
d. Fluid balance must be controlled carefully so that intake is limited to urine output plus insensible loss.
e. Seizures may be treated with slow IV infusion of diazepam (Valium), 0.2 mg/kg, or other anticonvulsant medication.
f. When a hypertensive crisis is under control, oral medications replace the parenteral medications (see Chapter 9, "Cardiovascular Drug Dosage").

HYPERLIPIDEMIA IN CHILDHOOD

A clear relationship has been established between elevated serum cholesterol levels and increased risk for coronary heart disease in adults. It is widely believed that atherosclerotic lesions start to develop in childhood and progress to irreversible lesions in adulthood. Therefore efforts to lower serum cholesterol levels in children have been made in the hope of preventing or retarding the progress of atherosclerosis. Reduction of elevated lipids is only one aspect of the total management plan. Other interrelated factors, such as genetics, hypertension, diabetes mellitus, obesity, and smoking, are important risk factors in the development of atherosclerotic cardiovascular disease. Physicians should play an increasing role not only in the detection of hyperlipidemia but in counseling for prevention of other risk factors.

Classification and Clinical Manifestations:

Brief outlines of each of the five types of hyperlipoproteinemia are presented in Figure 7–1. In childhood, hypercholesterolemia is usually a manifestation of an increased amount of LDL cholesterol (type II hyperlipoproteinemia). In this type the triglyceride levels are usually normal (type IIa), but are occasionally elevated (type IIb). Some children with abnormally high plasma cholesterol levels have concentrations of LDL cholesterol in the normal range, and above average or high HDL cholesterol levels. High levels of HDL are thought to be protec-

Types	Lipoproteins elevated	Lipids elevated	Prevalence in childhood	Symptoms and Signs	Treatment
Type I	Chylomicrons	Triglyceride (2000-4000 mg/dl)	Rare	Childhood onset (70%) Abdominal pain (pancreatitis) Eruptive exanthemas No coronary heart dis.	Low fat diet (10-15 gm/day)
Type IIa	LDL	Cholesterol	Common	Childhood or adulthood onset. Xanthomas of eyelids and palms. Achilles tendinitis Arcus cornea Coronary heart disease common in homozygotes	Diet (low cholesterol and high unsaturated fat) Cholestyramine, if not responsive to diet alone Weight loss if obese
Type IIb	LDL & VLDL	Cholesterol Triglyceride	Uncommon		
Type III	LDL & VLDL	Cholesterol Triglyceride	Very rare	Xanthomas; palmar and tuberosum Coronary heart dis (±)	Low fat and cholesterol diet Weight control Clofibrate?
Type IV	VLDL	Triglyceride	Relatively uncommon	Obesity Eruptive xanthomas Abdominal pain	Low fat and cholesterol diet Weight control
Type V	VLDL	Triglyceride Cholesterol (±)	Very rare	Obesity Eruptive xanthomas Coronary heart disease not frequent.	Low fat diet Weight control

FIG 7–1.
Summary of clinical features of hyperlipoproteinemia. (Modified from Park MK: *Pediatric Cardiology for Practitioners*, ed 2. Chicago, Year Book Medical Publishers, 1988.)

tive against atherosclerosis. It is therefore important to determine HDL cholesterol levels in children with hypercholesterolemia to distinguish those with type II hyperlipoproteinemia from those with normal LDL cholesterol levels.

Elevated plasma levels of lipids or lipoproteins may be primary or secondary. The primary form is genetically determined. The secondary form may result from diets high in cholesterol and saturated fat, from a variety of disease states (e.g., liver disease, lupus, hypothyroidism, diabetes mellitus, nephrotic syndrome), or from other causes (oral contraceptives, alcohol, steroids).

Prevention of Childhood Hyperlipidemia

The American Health Foundation recommends the following screening, verification, and management strategies for pediatric hyperlipidemia (*Prev Med* 1989; 18: 323–409):

1. Screen all children any time after age 2 years for baseline total cholesterol (TC). If TC is less than 175 mg/dL (75th percentile), repeat in 3–5 years.
2. If TC is greater than 175 mg/dL, if a family history (FH) is positive for premature coronary heart disease or hyperlipidemia, or if other risk factors are present, perform a lipoprotein profile (TC, HDL-C, LDL-C, triglyceride [TG]). The level of LDL-C can be calculated using the Friedewall formula so long as TG levels are 400 mg/dL or lower.

$$\text{LDL-C} = \text{TC} - (\text{TG}/5 + \text{HDL-C})$$

3. Based on TC and LDL-C levels, children are divided into four groups: (a) low risk (TC <175 mg/dL); (b) moderate risk (TC 175–200 mg/dL, LDL-C 110–140 mg/dL); (c) high risk (TC >200 mg/dL, LDL-C >140 mg/dL); (d) very high risk (TC >230 mg/dL, LDL-C >160 mg/dL).
4. Management of each group:
   a. Low risk: Routine care. Nutrition counseling (AHA step 1 diet, physical activity, no smoking).

Repeat screen in 3–5 years.

b. Moderate risk: Routine care (same as for low risk group). Nutritional counseling. Rule out secondary hyperlipidemia. Consider family screening.
c. High risk: Routine care. AHA step 2 diet after 3 months on step 1 diet if TC and LDL-C are not lower. Family nutrition counseling. Rule out secondary hyperlipidemia. Consider family screening.
d. Very high risk: Routine care. AHA step 2 diet after 3–4 months on step 1 diet if cholesterol levels are not lower. Family screening and counseling. Consider referral to a lipid specialist. Consider drug therapy if levels are still high after 6–12 months.

MANAGEMENT OF SURGICAL PATIENTS VIII

J. H. Calhoon, D. Rasch, D-H. Lee, and M. K. Park

Cardiac surgery in the newborn, infant, and child is divided into two types of procedures; open-heart procedures and closed procedures. Open-heart procedures utilize cardiopulmonary bypass (CPB) with cardiac arrest and some degree of hypothermia, with or without circulatory arrest. Open procedures are required for repair of intracardiac anomalies (e.g., VSD, TOF, TGA). Closed procedures do not require CPB and are performed for repair of extracardiac anomalies (e.g., COA, PDA) or palliative procedures (S-P procedures or PA banding).

The current trend is to carry out total repair of CHD at an early age, whenever such repair is technically possible. This approach is made possible by improved surgical technique and better understanding of postoperative intensive care of newborns and small infants. Early total repair negates the need for palliative procedures and possibly prevents permanent damage to the cardiovascular system, which is known to develop in certain CHDs. Recommendations for early repair of CHD in the neonate or small infant are made on an individual basis in a joint cardiology–cardiac surgery conference; the indications vary among institutions.

In the following sections we outline some pertinent aspects of preoperative management and postoperative care of cardiac patients.

I. PREOPERATIVE MANAGEMENT OF CARDIAC PATIENTS

1. Regular diet (limited fluid and salt intake in CHF).
2. Laboratory evaluation:
   a. CBC, platelet count, PT, PTT.
   b. Type and cross-match 2–4 units packed RBCs, and platelets, 6 units/m^2, for cyanotic infants.
   c. Serum electrolytes, BUN, glucose, and creatinine.
   d. CXR and ECG.
   e. Urinalysis.
3. Medications:
   a. Digoxin is discontinued after the evening dose.
   b. Diuretics are discontinued 8–12 hours preoperatively (or this must be individualized).
   c. Propranolol and antiarrhythmics are continued at the same dosage until immediately before the surgery.
   d. Patients who have received long-term steroid therapy receive steroids in the preoperative period.
   e. Nonsteroidal anti-inflammatory drugs (aspirin, indomethacin, ibuprofen [Motrin]) and antiplatelet drugs (dipyridamole [Persantine], sulfinpyrazone [Anturane]) should be discontinued 7 or more days before surgery (because of the platelet inhibiting action).
4. Preoperative antibiotics:
   Cephalosporin (Ancef or equivalent), 75–100 mg/kg/day IV, immediately before surgery. (Continued every 8 hours after surgery for 3 days or until chest tubes are removed).

II. POSTOPERATIVE CARE OF CARDIAC PATIENTS

Postoperative care of cardiac patients can be simplified by a systems approach, that is, looking at the patient systematically from cardiovascular, pulmonary, renal, metabolic, hematologic, and CNS points of view.

A. Normal Convalescence:

Normally convalescing postoperative cardiac patients should have the following findings, according to the systems approach:

1. Cardiovascular system: Cardiac output, BP, and heart rate should be normal, and sinus rhythm should be present.
   a. Skin should be warm to the touch over the extremities, and good pedal pulses with brisk capillary refill should be present. Normal BP and adequate urine output (at least 1 mL/kg/hr) are clinical evidence of good cardiac output. Measured cardiac index by thermodilution method should be greater than 2.0 L/min/m^2.
   b. Mild arterial hypertension is present in the early postoperative period following CPB (because of a high SVR resulting from increased levels of catecholamines, plasma renin, or angiotensin II).
   c. Heart rate is relatively high (>100 beats/min in infants and >80 beats/min in older children), and the rhythm should be sinus.
2. Pulmonary system:
   a. Normal arterial blood gases and pH.
   b. CXRs should show no evidence of pneumothorax, atelectasis, or pleural effusion, and the ET tube and chest tubes should be in acceptable positions.
3. Renal system:
   a. Adequate urine output (>1 mL/kg/hr).
   b. Evidence of adequate solute excretion (Serum

K <5 mEq/L, BUN <40 mg/dL, creatinine <1.0 mg/dL).

4. Metabolic system:
   a. Retention of water and sodium and depletion of whole-body potassium are commonly seen following CPB, resulting in mild hyponatremia and hypokalemia and 5% weight gain.
   b. Mild metabolic acidosis (base deficit ≤4 mEq/L) is common in the first few hours after CPB and does not require treatment.
   c. Normal serum calcium and absence of hypoglycemia.
   d. Varying degree of fever (temperature up to 39.5° C) is nearly always present during the first 4–5 days, and extensive workup for infection is not indicated. History and physical examination should always be performed again to rule out a correctable cause. Causes of fever include reaction to CPB, infection, reaction to homologous blood, atelectasis, pleural effusion, low cardiac output, and brain stem damage.
5. Hematologic system:
   a. Blood balance should be maintained according to the I & O sheet.
   b. Normal clotting studies and hemoglobin >9.5 gm/dL.
6. Neurologic system:
   a. Responses appropriate for level of sedation.
   b. Absence of neurologic defects (hemiplegia, visual field defects) or seizures.

B. Abnormal Convalescence:

The following findings suggest abnormal convalescence, and need to be monitored and treated.

1. Cardiovascular system.
   a. Inadequate cardiac output is diagnosed when the following are present.
      (a) Cold extremities and weak pulses.
      (b) Oliguria (urine output <1 mL/kg/hr).

(c) Rising serum K levels (to 5 mEq/L).
(d) P_{VO_2} from RA or central venous line <28 mm Hg.
(e) Measured cardiac index <2.0 L/min/m^2.

Causes of and treatment for low cardiac output:

(1) Low preload: It is treated with increase in blood volume to raise atrial pressure to 15–20 mm Hg.
(2) High afterload: Vasodilators or morphine infusion.
(3) Incomplete or inadequate surgical repair (such as R–L shunt or residual L–R shunt). Can be detected by Echo and Doppler studies or cardiac catheterization. Immediate surgical repair is occasionally indicated.
(4) Cardiac tamponade: Detected by Echo. Decompression of pericardial space is indicated.
(5) Depressed myocardial function may be treated by:
    (a) Dopamine starting at 2.5 μg/kg/min and increasing up to 15 μg/kg/min if necessary.
    (b) Epinephrine, isoproterenal, or dobutamine may be gradually added in similar dosage if dopamine is not effective.
    (c) Digitalis is not given in the first 24–48 hours because of (a) frequent occurrence of hypokalemia, which potentiates digitalis toxicity, (b) unstable renal function, and (c) CPB-sensitized myocardium prone to digitalis toxicity.
(6) Other measures that aid in correction of low cardiac output include:
    (a) Raising heart rate to optimum by atrial or ventricular pacing or chronotropic agents. Atrial and ventricular pacing wires are routinely placed dur-

ing surgery and are left for 5–7 days postoperatively.

(b) Optimize hemoglobin to 12–14 gm/dL (at least higher than 9.5 gm/dL).

(c) Raise Pao_2 to 100–200 mm Hg by increasing Fio_2 or increasing ventilation.

(d) Sedation or paralyzing drugs to prevent restlessness or agitation (which increase O_2 consumption).

(e) Narcotic infusion with or without paralyzing agents in infants with pulmonary hypertension to prevent paroxysms of pulmonary vasospasm.

b. Hypotension or hypertension:

(1) Treat hypotension if BP drops to the lower ranges of normal with volume expanders, initially 10–20 mL/kg. If this fails, treat with inotropic agents. (Remember that citrated blood products bind ionized Ca, and $CaCl_2$ may be helpful).

(2) Although mild hypertension in the early postoperative period is common, severe hypertension is treated with vasodilators.

c. Rhythm disorders:

Sinus rhythm is the optimal rhythm. Nodal (or AV junctional) rhythm may reduce cardiac output by 10% to 15%. Certain atrial arrhythmias and most ventricular arrhythmias should be investigated and treated. Evaluate oxygenation, ventilator function, acid base status, serum K, and dosages of cardiotonic agents.

(1) Frequent PVCs (more than six per minute) are treated with lidocaine, 1 mg/kg IV.

(2) Ventricular tachycardia is treated with lidocaine, DC cardioversion, or overdrive suppression.

(3) Atrial fibrillation is treated with digoxin with or without cardioversion.

(4) Atrial flutter is treated with overdrive sup-

pression and digoxin (for 8 weeks) to prevent recurrences.

(5) SVT is treated with overdrive suppression or cardioversion. Cautious use of propranolol or verapamil IV. Digoxin for 8 weeks to prevent recurrences.

d. Bradycardia or tachycardia:
Bradycardia and extreme tachycardia decrease cardiac output. Ranges of heart rate in normally convalescing patients are as follows:

<6 mo	110–190
6–12 mo	100–170
1–3 yr	90–160
>3 yr	80–150

(1) Bradycardia is treated by atrial or ventricular pacing or chronotropic agents.

(2) Tachycardia may be caused by fever, volume depletion, or arrhythmias. Treatment should be directed to the correction of causes.

2. Pulmonary system:
   a. Abnormal blood gases: Abnormal $Paco_2$ is corrected by changing the ventilator rate or volume. Low Pao_2 is corrected by raising Fio_2, adding PEEP, or increasing tidal volume.
   b. Significant degrees of pneumothorax or pleural effusion may require treatment.
   c. An unacceptable ET tube position requires correction. Ideally, the tip of the ET tube should be 2–3 cm above the carina.
   d. Increasing width of the mediastinal shadow suggests accumulation of blood. (Investigate function of the mediastinal chest tube.)
   e. Respiratory settings: The rate and depth of respirations should be adjusted to maintain acceptable Pao_2 and $Paco_2$. PEEP 3–5 cm. H_2O is used in children. PEEP is contraindicated following Senning's operation, Fontan's operation, or Glenn's operation (to avoid high jugular venous pressure).

f. Extubation is performed as soon as possible, usually in the operating room in children undergoing closed operations, within 4–8 hours following uncomplicated open heart procedures, and the following morning after complex open procedures.
   Criteria for extubation:
   (1) Patient awake and alert.
   (2) Satisfactory hemodynamic state (normal BP, adequate cardiac output, no significant arrhythmias).
   (3) Absence of important bleeding (minimal chest tube drainage).
   (4) Arterial Po_2 >100 mm Hg with ventilator rate of 6/min and Fio_2 0.40.
   (5) Spontaneous respiratory rate of 40/min in young children and 50/min in infants.
   (6) Absence of use of accessory respiratory muscle.
   (7) Normal $Paco_2$ and pH.

3. Renal system:
   a. Acute renal failure:
      Oliguria (<1 mL/kg/hr) and evidence of solute accumulation (serum K >5 mEq/L, BUN >40 mg/dL, creatinine >1.0 mg/dL) indicate acute renal failure. Acute reduction of cardiac output is the most common cause of renal failure. It occurs more frequently in cyanotic infants after a prolonged period of CPB and in patients with postoperative hemolysis.
      (1) Initial treatment is directed to improving cardiac output and inducing diuresis.
         (a) Optimize preload and afterload (see above).
         (b) Dopamine infusion.
         (c) Lasix, 1 mg/kg IV. If no response, 2 mg/kg, then 4 mg/kg. May be repeated every 6–12 hours for 3 days.
      (2) If serum K >6.5 mEq/L, glucose-insulin solution (0.5 gm glucose/kg with 0.3 U crystalline insulin/gm glucose, IV over 2

hours) and K-exalate enema are given.

(3) Peritoneal dialysis may be necessary.

4. Metabolic system:

a. Fluid replacement: Because of the tendency to retain Na and water, a minimal amount of dextrose in water (D5W in infants, D10W in children) without Na is administered for approximately 48 hours after operation. A modest amount of K (10 mEq/m^2/day) is given on the first day after operation. Recommended fluid volume replacements in the first 24 hours after open or closed procedures are as follows:

60 mL/kg for first 10 kg body weight (BW)
30 mL/kg for second 10 kg BW
15 mL/kg for remainder of BW

b. Abnormalities of electrolytes and acid-base balance:

(1) Mild hyponatremia does not require treatment other than fluid restriction and diuretics. Serum Na <125 mEq/L requires treatment to elevate Na levels.

(2) Hypernatremia with serum Na >155 mEq/L needs to be treated with Na restriction and liberalization of fluids.

(3) Treat metabolic acidosis if the base deficit is >−5 mEq/L. Total extracellular base deficit = base deficit (mEq/L) × 0.3 × BW (kg).

The dosage of $NaHCO_3$ is half of the total extracellular base deficit.

c. Treat hypoglycemia (<50 mg/dL) or hypocalcemia.

d. Fever (temperature >38.5° C):

(1) Acetaminophen suppository, 10 mg/kg, every 4 hours (aspirin not used).

(2) Dexamethasone, 0.25 mg/kg IV, then 0.1 mg/kg IV every 6 hours for four doses (for possible transfusion reaction).

(3) Cooling blanket if temperature >39.8° C

and fever not responding to acetaminophen.
(4) Na nitroprusside to increase peripheral heat loss.
(5) Pancuronium to reduce muscle heat production.

e. Nutrition: Oral feeding is begun in infants 8 hours after extubation, starting with glucose water every 4 hours and advancing to an appropriate formula. Gavage feeding if infant is too weak to suck. In infants with prolonged intubation, gavage feeding or TPN is required.

5. Hematologic system and volume infusion:
   a. Correct anemia and maintain a desirable filling pressure (LA pressure 6–14 mm Hg) by infusion of either packed RBCs, salt-poor albumin, or plasma, depending on hemoglobin level or hematocrit.
      (1) Children: Packed RBCs if Hgb <10 gm/dL (or Hct $<30\%$); colloid solution if Hgb >10 gm/dL (or Hct $>30\%$).
      (2) Maintain Hct $>45\%$ in newborns, 35–40% in small infants.
   b. Necessity to infuse more than 10–15 mL/kg volume requires investigation for excessive blood loss and for possible surgical reentry into the chest cavity to control bleeding.
   c. Correct coagulation abnormalities.
6. Neurologic system:
   a. Localized neurologic defects such as hemiplegia and visual field defects are abnormal; may be due to air or particulate emboli.
   b. Seizures may be caused by metabolic abnormalities, infections, cerebral edema, embolism or hemorrhage, or decreased cerebral perfusion. Seizures seldom have ominous long-term complications. Management of seizures includes the following:
      (1) Determine arterial blood gases; serum glu-

cose, Ca, and electrolytes; cardiac output; and temperature. Correct any abnormalities.

(2) Anticonvulsant therapy:
   (a) Diazepam (Valium), 0.1–0.2 mg/kg IV, if assisted ventilation used. (Diazepam has respiratory depressant effects.)
   (b) Phenobarbital, 10–15 mg/kg IV over 5–10 minutes. (Full effect may take several hours.)
   (c) Phenytoin (Dilantin), 20 mg/kg PO, followed by a maintenance dose of 3–4 mg/kg/day PO.
   (d) Phenobarbital maintenance: 2.5 mg/kg/dose twice daily.

c. Choreiform movement and grossly inadequate behavior are more major neurologic complications. Pharmacologic control is difficult. These complications usually, but not always, clear without demonstrable sequelae.

C. Postoperative Orders:

The following is an example of postoperative orders for cardiac patients:

1. Vital signs every 20 minutes until stable, then ICU routine.
2. NPO; NG tube to low wall suction; irrigate as necessary with NS; chest tube to 10 cm H_2O, Foley catheter to gravity.
3. Record I & O every hour.
4. CXR and ECG on admission and in morning.
5. CBC, platelet count, serum electrolytes, glucose, calcium, and arterial blood gases in 20 minutes.
6. Arterial blood gases, serum K, hematocrit every 4–8 hours first day, then as desirable. In infants younger than 1 year, check serum Ca and glucose levels every 4–8 hours the first day, then as desirable.

7. Arterial lines: NS with 1 U heparin/mL at 2 mL/hr. Intracardiac lines: D5 1/4NS with 1 U heparin/mL at 2 mL/hr.
8. IV fluid: D51/4NS (infants D101/4NS) with 10 mEq KCl/500 mL to run at ___ mL/hr for first 24 hours.
9. Keep preload optimal with either packed RBCs, Plasmanate, or FFP.
10. Ventilator settings begin at F_{IO_2} 1.0 initially, and may be reduced when arterial blood gas values are available. The lowest F_{IO_2} for first 24 hours is 0.4. Make ventilator changes in one category at a time (i.e., F_{IO_2}, peak pressure, tidal volume, rate). Arterial blood gas values should be sent within 15–20 minutes of any ventilator changes.
11. Medications:
    a. Cefazolin (Ancef), 25–30 mg/kg IV every 8 hours.
    b. Morphine sulfate, 0.1 mg/kg IV every 2–4 hours.
    c. Diazepam (Valium), 0.1 mg/kg every 3–4 hours as necessary.
    d. Chloral hydrate, 50–75 mg/kg/dose PO or PR every 6 hours as necessary.
    e. KCl, 0.5 mEq/kg IV bolus over 1 minute as necessary for K^+ <4 mEq/L.
    f. Furosemide (Lasix), 1 mg/kg IV every 8 hours.
    g. Dopamine, 2–5 μg/kg/min IV drip.
    h. Maalox, 2–5 mL for infants, 5–12 mL for children, every 2 hours through NG tube, as necessary for pH <5.

III. POSTOPERATIVE SYNDROMES

Four well-recognized syndromes are seen in the period following heart surgery in children.

A. Postcoarctectomy Syndrome:

This syndrome is believed to be caused by arteritis resulting from changes in pressure and flow dynamics following resection of the COA. The arteritis most often involves the superior mesenteric artery distribution. The syndrome is characterized by severe intermittent abdominal pain, fever, and leukocytosis, mimicking acute surgical abdomen, occurring 2–8 days after the surgery. In severe cases abdominal distention, melena, and ascites associated with gangrenous bowel may develop. Rebound systemic hypertension may be present.

Careful monitoring of BP and prevention of rebound hypertension is important, by administration of β-adrenergic blockers (e.g., propranolol), vasodilators (e.g., hydralazine), and sympatholytic drugs (e.g., reserpine).

B. Postpericardiotomy Syndrome:

This syndrome is believed to represent an immunologic phenomenon as a sequela of blood in the pericardial sac. The onset of the syndrome is 2–3 weeks after surgery that involves pericardiotomy. It is rare in infants younger than 2 years of age. The syndrome is characterized by fever (sustained or spiking; temperature to 103° F [39.4° C]), chest pain, pericardial friction rub, pericardial and pleural effusion, and hepatomegaly. Leukocytosis with shift to the left and elevated ESR are present. CXRs show enlarged cardiac silhouette; ECG shows persistent ST and T changes; Echo shows pericardial effusion or signs of cardiac tamponade.

Bed rest is all that is needed in mild cases (it subsides in 2–3 weeks). Aspirin may be used for chest pain, and moderate doses of corticosteroids for a few days may be indicated in severe cases. Pericardial window is indicated for signs of cardiac tamponade (uncommon). Diuretics may be used for pleural effusion.

C. Postperfusion Syndrome:

Postperfusion syndrome after open-heart surgery using CPB is believed to be due to cytomegalovirus infection. The syndrome occurs 3–6 weeks after surgery and is characterized by the triad of fever (temperature up to 103° F [39.4° C]), splenomegaly (lasting for 8 weeks), and atypical lymphocytosis (lasting 2–3 weeks). No specific treatment is available. The syndrome is self-limited, lasting for a few weeks to a few months.

D. Hemolytic Anemia Syndrome:

Hemolytic anemia may occur after cardiac surgery, especially repair of ECD or aortic or mitral valve replacement. It is caused by trauma of red blood cells or by autoimmune reaction.

The syndrome occurs 1–2 weeks after the surgery and is characterized by low-grade fever, jaundice, hepatomegaly, and reticulocytosis. Medical treatment consists of iron replacement therapy or blood transfusion. Surgical correction of turbulence is indicated if the anemia is severe.

CARDIOVASCULAR DRUG DOSAGE IX

Drug dosages listed in this chapter are derived from several sources. *Physicians' Desk Reference* (PDR), *The Pediatric Drug Handbook* (Benitz and Tatro), and *The Harriet Lane Handbook* are the primary sources of drug dosage. Less frequently used include tables developed by Levine and Zenk, by Hurwitz, and by Park, and journal articles.

1. *Physicians' Desk Reference,* ed 44. Oradell, NJ, Medical Economics Co, 1990.
2. Benitz WE, Tatro DS: *The Pediatric Drug Handbook,* ed 2. Chicago, Year Book Medical Publishers, 1988.
3. Cole CH: *The Harriet Lane Handbook,* ed 10. Chicago, Year Book Medical Publishers, 1984.
4. Levin RH, Zenk KE: Medication table, in Rudolph AM, Hoffman JIE (eds): *Pediatrics,* ed 18. Norwalk, Conn, Appleton and Lange, 1987, pp 1839–1867.
5. Hurwitz RA: Drugs and dosages in pediatrics, in Adams FH, Emmanouilides GC, Reimenschneider TA (eds): *Moss' Heart Disease in Infants and Children,* ed 4. Baltimore, Williams & Wilkins, 1989, pp 1038–1048.
6. Park MK: *Pediatric Cardiology for Practitioners,* ed 2. Chicago, Year Book Medical Publishers, 1988.

FORMULARY

Drug	Route and Dosage	Toxicity or Side Effects	How Supplied
A. Cardiac Glycosides			
Digoxin (Lanoxin)	**Children:** *Total digitalizing dose (TDD):* (PO): Premature 20 μg/kg Full-term newborn 30 μg/kg 1 mo–2 yr 40–50 μg/kg >2 yr 30–40 μg/kg (IV) 75%–80% of PO dose *Maintenance dose:* (PO, IV): 25%–30% of TDD/day in 2 doses	AV conduction disturbances, arrhythmias, nausea/vomiting (see Table 7–4 for ECG signs)	Elixir: 50 μg/mL (60 mL) Tab: 0.125, 0.25, 0.5 mg Inj: 100, 250 μg/mL
Digitoxin (Crystodigin, Digitaline Nativelle, Purodigin)	**Children:** *Total digitalizing dose (TDD):* (PO) Premature and full-term newborn 20 μg/kg 1 mo–2 yr 30 μg/kg >2 yr 20 μg/kg (IV,IM): Same as PO TDD *Maintenance dose:* (PO,IV,IM): 15% (10%–20%) of TDD once a day	Same as for digoxin	Elixir: Digitaline Nativelle 50 μg/mL Tab: 0.05, 0.1 mg Inj: 0.2 mg/mL

B. Inotropic Agents

Amrinone* (Inocor) (non-catecholamine inotropic agent with vasodilator effects)	**Children:** (IV): *Loading:* 0.5 mg/kg over 2–3 min in 1/2NS (not D5W) *Maintenance:* 5–20 μg/kg/min **Adults:** (IV): *Loading:* 0.75 mg/kg over 2–3 min *Maintenance:* 5–10 μg/kg/min	Hypotension, tachyarrhythmias, thrombocytopenia, nausea/vomiting, hepatotoxicity, fever	Inj: 5 mg/mL (20 mL)
Dobutamine (Dobutrex) (β_1-adrenergic stimulator)	**Children:** (IV): 2–15 μg/kg/min in D5W or NS (incompatible with alkali solution) **Adults:** (IV): 2.5–10.0 μg/kg/min	Tachyarrhythmias, hypertension, nausea/vomiting, headache (Contraindicated in IHSS and atrial flutter/fibrillation)	Inj: 12.5 mg/mL (20 mL vial)
Dopamine (Intropin, Dopastat)	Effects are dose dependent: (a) 2–5 μg/kg/min ↑ Renal blood flow (RBF) and urine output (b) 5–15 μg/kg/min ↑ RBF, ↑ heart rate (HR), ↑ cardiac contractility and cardiac output	Tachyarrhythmias, nausea/vomiting, hypotension or hypertension, extravasation (tissue necrosis; treat with local infiltration of phentolamine)	Inj: 40 mg/mL (5 mL) 80 mg/mL (5 mL) 160 mg/mL (5 mL)

**Not yet approved or not enough information available for pediatric dosage.*

(Continued.)

Drug	Route and Dosage	Toxicity or Side Effects	How Supplied
	(c) >20 μg/kg/min α-Adrenergic effects with ↓ RBF(±) (Incompatible with alkali solution)		
Epinephrine (Adrenalin) (α-, β_1-, β_2-adrenergic stimulator)	**Children:** (IV): 1:10,000 solution Begin with 0.1 μg/kg/min; increase to 1 μg/kg/min to achieve desired effects	Tachyarrhythmias, hypertension, nausea/vomiting, headache, tissue necrosis(±)	Inj: 0.01 mg/mL (1:100,000 solution: 5 mL) 0.1 mg/mL (1:10,000 solution: 10 mL) 1 mg/mL (1:1,000 solution: 1 mL)
Isoproterenol (Isuprel) (β_1-, β_2-adrenergic stimulator)	**Children:** (IV): 0.1–1.5 μg/kg/min; titrate to desired effect **Adults:** (IV): 2–20 μg/min; titrate to desired effect (Incompatible with alkali solution)	Similar as for epinephrine	Inj: 0.2 mg/mL (1:5,000 solution: 1, 5 mL)
Milrinone* (phosphodiesterase inhibitor)	**Children:** (IV): 0.01–0.05 μg/kg/dose, then 0.1–1.0 μg/kg/min	Renal dysfunction, arrhythmias	Inj: 1 mg/mL

C. Diuretics			
Acetazolamide (Diamox)	**Children:** (PO,IV): 5.0 mg/kg/dose once a day or once every other day **Adults:** (PO,IV): 250–375 mg/dose once a day or once every other day	Paresthesia, GI irritation, anorexia, drowsiness, fatigue, transient hypokalemia, reduced uric acid excretion	Tab: 125, 250 mg Inj: 500 mg/5 mL
Chlorothiazide (Diuril)	**Children:** (PO): 20–40 mg/kg/day in 2 doses **Adults:** (PO): 250–500 mg/dose once a day or intermittently	Hypokalemia, hyponatremia, hypochloremic alkalosis, prerenal azotemia, hyperuricemia, hyperglycemia, rarely blood dyscrasias, allergic reactions	PO susp: 250 mg/5 mL (237 mL) Tab: 250, 500 mg Inj: 500 mg (vial, for reconstruction with 18 mL sterile water)
Ethacrynic acid (Edecrin)	**Children:** (PO): 25 mg/dose once a day (max 2–3 mg/kg/day) (IV): 1 mg/kg/dose **Adults:** (PO): 50–100 mg once a day (max 400 mg/day) (IV): 0.5–1 mg/kg/dose or 50 mg/dose	Dehydration, hypokalemia prerenal azotemia, hyperuricemia, 8th cranial nerve damage (deafness), abnormal LFT, agranulocytosis or thrombocytopenia, GI irritation, rash	Tab: 25, 50 mg Inj: 50 mg (vial, for reconstruction with 50 mL D5W)

*Not yet approved or not enough information available for pediatric dosage.

(Continued.)

FORMULARY (cont.)

Drug	Route and Dosage	Toxicity or Side Effects	How Supplied
Furosemide (Lasix)	**Children:** (IV): 0.5–2 mg/kg/dose 2–4 times/day (Max 6 mg/kg/dose) (PO): 1–2 mg/kg/dose 2–3 times/day prn **Adults:** (IV): 20–40 mg/dose 2–4 times/day (PO): 20–80 mg/dose 3–4 times/day prn	Hypokalemia, hyperuricemia, prerenal azotemia, ototoxicity, rarely blood dyscrasias, rash	PO sol: 10 mg/mL (60 mL) Tab: 20, 40, 80 mg Inj: 10 mg/mL (2, 4, 10 mL)
Hydrochloro-thiazide (HydroDiuril)	**Children:** (PO): 2–4 mg/kg/day in 2 doses **Adults:** (PO): 25–100 mg/dose once a day or intermittently	Same as for chlorothiazide	Tab: 25, 50, 100 mg
Spironolactone (Aldactone)	**Children:** (PO): 2–3 mg/kd/day in 2–3 doses **Adults:** (PO): 25–100 mg/day in 2–4 doses (max 200 mg/day)	Hyperkalemia (with K supplements)	Tab: 25, 50, 100 mg

Triamterene (Dyrenium)	**Children:** (PO): 2–4 mg/kg/day in 1–2 doses **Adults:** (PO): 100–300 mg/day in 1–2 doses (max 300 mg/day)	Nausea/vomiting, leg cramps, dizziness, hyperuricemia, rash	Caps: 50, 100 mg
D. Vasopressor Agents			
Ephedrine sulfate (α-, β-adrenoreceptor stimulant)	**Children:** (IV,IM): 0.2–0.3 mg/kg/dose q4–6h prn **Adults:** (IV): 5–25 mg/dose q3–4h (IM,SC): 25–50 mg/dose q4–6h	Similar as for epinephrine	Inj: 25, 50 mg/mL
Norepinephrine (Levophed, Levarterenol) (α-, β-adrenoreceptor stimulant)	**Children:** (IV): 0.1 μg/kg/min initially; increase dose to attain desired effects **Adults:** (IV): Add 4 mL Levophed to 1,000 mL D5W; start at 2–3 mL (8–12 μg)/min and adjust rate	Hypertension, bradycardia (reflex), arrhythmias, tissue necrosis (treat with phentolamine infiltration)	Inj: 1 mg/mL
Metaraminol (Aramine) (α-, β-adrenoreceptor stimulant)	**Children:** (IV): 0.01 mg/kg/dose IV bolus 5 μg/kg/min IV infusion initially; titrate to achieve desired effects	Similar as for norepinephrine	Inj: 10 mg/mL

(Continued.)

Drug	Route and Dosage	Toxicity or Side Effects	How Supplied
	Adults: (IV): 0.5–5 mg IV bolus q5–10 min prn 1–4 μg/kg/min IV infusion		
Phenylephrine (Neo-Synephrine) (α-adrenoceptor stimulant)	For *hypotension:* **Children** (IM,SC): 0.1 mg/kg/dose q1–2h prn (IV): 5–10 μg/kg/dose IV bolus q10–15 min 0.1–0.5 μg/kg/min IV infusion **Adults:** (IV): 0.1–0.5 mg/dose IV bolus q10–15 min prn Start infusion at 100–180 μg/min; maintain at 40–60 μg/min	Arrhythmias, hypertension, angina	Inj: 10 mg/mL

E. Antihypertensive and Vasodilatory Agents

Drug	Route and Dosage	Toxicity or Side Effects	How Supplied
Atenolol* (Tenormin) (β-adrenoreceptor blocker)	**Children:** (PO): 1–2 mg/kg/day once a day **Adults:** (PO): 50 mg once a day for 1–2 wk (alone or with diuretic) May increase to 100 mg once a day	CNS symptoms (dizziness, tiredness, depression), rash, nausea/vomiting, blood dyscrasias (agranulocytosis, purpura)	Tab: 50, 100 mg

Captopril (Capoten) (angiotensin I converting enzyme inhibitor)	**Children:** (PO): <6 mo: 0.05–0.5 mg/kg 3 times/day >6 mo: 0.5–2.0 mg/kg 3 times/day (Max 6 mg/kg/day) **Adults:** (PO): 25 mg 2–3 times/day initially Increase to 50 mg 2–3 times/day q1–2 wk (max 150 mg 3 times/day) (Usually used with diuretic)	Neutropenia/agranulocytosis, proteinuria, hypotension and tachycardia, rash, taste impairment	Tab: 12.5, 25, 50, 100 mg
Chlorothiazide Ethacrynic acid Furosemide Hydrochlorothiazide	(See "Diuretics")		
Diazoxide (Hyperstat) (peripheral vasodilator)	*For emergencies:* **Children/Adults** (IV): 1–3 mg/kg (max 150 mg single dose) repeated q15min; titrate to desired effects	Hypotension, hyperglycemia, nausea/vomiting, Na retention (CHF±)	Inj: 15 mg/mL

**Not yet approved or not enough information available for pediatric dosage.*

(Continued.)

Drug	Route and Dosage	Toxicity or Side Effects	How Supplied
Hydralazine (Apresoline) (peripheral vasodilator)	**Children:** (IM,IV): 0.15–0.2 mg/kg/dose (for emergency) May be repeated q4–6h (PO) 0.75–3 mg/kg/day in 2–4 doses **Adults:** (IM,IV): 10–50 mg/dose (for emergency) (PO): Start with 10 mg 4 times/day for 2–4 days Increase to 25 mg 4 times/day for 3–4 days, then to 50 mg 4 times/day	Hypotension, tachycardia and palpitation, lupus-like syndrome with prolonged use (fever, arthralgia, splenomegaly and +LE prep), blood dyscrasias (rare)	Inj: 20 mg/mL Tab: 10, 25, 50, 100 mg
Minoxidil (Loniten) (peripheral vasodilator)	**Children** <12 yr: (PO): 0.2 mg/kg once a day initially May be increased in 50%–100% increments Usual dose: 0.25–1.0 mg/kg/day in 1–2 doses (Max 50 mg/day)	Reflex tachycardia and fluid retention (used with a beta blocker and diuretic), pericardial effusion, hypertrichosis, blood dyscrasias (rarely leukopenia, thrombocytopenia)	Tab: 2.5, 10 mg

	Children >12 yr and Adults: (PO): 5 mg once a day initially May be increased to 10, 20, 40 mg in single or divided doses Usual dose 10–40 mg/day (max 100 mg/day)		
Methyldopa (Aldomet)	**Children:** (IV): 5–10 mg/kg/dose over 30–60 min, then 20–40 mg/kg/day in 4 doses (max 65 mg/kg/day or 3 g/day) (PO): 10 mg/kg/day in 2–4 doses May be increased or decreased (max 65 mg/kg/day or 3 g/day) **Adults:** (IV): 250–500 mg q6h (max 1 g q6h) (PO): 250 mg 2–3 times/day for 2 days May be increased or decreased q2 days Usual dose 0.5–2 g/day in 2–4 doses (max 3 g/day)	Sedation, orthostatic hypotension and bradycardia, lupus-like syndrome, Coombs (+) hemolytic anemia and leukopenia, hepatitis/cirrhosis, colitis, impotence	Inj: 50 mg/mL PO susp: 250 mg/5 mL (16 oz) Tab: 125, 250, 500 mg

(Continued.)

FORMULARY (cont.)

Drug	Route and Dosage	Toxicity or Side Effects	How Supplied
Metoprolol* (Lopressor) (β-adrenoreceptor blocker)	**Children:** (PO): 1–5 mg/kg/day in 2 doses **Adults:** (PO): 100 mg/day in 1–3 doses initially May increase to 450 mg/day in 2–3 doses Usual dose 100–450 mg/day (Usually used with hydrochlorothiazide 25–100 mg/day)	CNS symptoms (dizziness, tiredness, depression), bronchospasm, bradycardia, diarrhea, nausea/vomiting, abdominal pain	Tab: 50, 100 mg
Nifedipine* (Procardia, Adalat) (Ca channel blocker)	**Children:** *For hypertrophic cardiomyopathy:* (PO): 0.6–0.9 mg/kg/day in 3–4 doses **Adults:** (PO): 10 mg 3 times/day initially Titrate up to 20 or 30 mg 3–4 times/day over 7–14 days Usual dose 10–20 mg 3 times/day (max 180 mg/day)	Hypotension, peripheral edema, CNS symptoms (headache, dizziness, weakness), nausea	Caps: 10 mg

Nitroprusside (Nipride) (peripheral vasodilator)	**Children:** (IV): 0.5–10 μg/kg/min, with BP monitoring Usual dose 2–3 μg/kg/min (Dilute stock solution [50 mg] in 250–1,000 mL D5W; light sensitive)	Hypotension, sweating and palpitations, nausea/vomiting, cyanide toxicity (metabolic acidosis the earliest and most reliable evidence; monitor thiocyanate level when used >48h and in renal failure)	Inj: 50 mg (vial, for reconstruction with 2–3 mL D5W)
Phentolamine (Regitine) (α-adrenoreceptor blocker)	*For pheochromocytoma:* (IM,IV): **Children,** 1 mg **Adults,** 5 mg 1–2h preoperatively and during surgery; repeated q2–4h prn for prevention/ treatment of hypertension *For treatment of extravasated drugs:* (SC): 0.1–0.2 mg/kg locally within 12h (max 10 mg)	Hypotension, tachycardia/arrhythmias, nausea/vomiting	Inj: 5 mg/mL
Prazosine* (Minipress) (postsynaptic α-adrenergic blocker)	**Children:** (PO): 5 μg/kg as a test dose, then 25–150 μg/kg/day in 4 doses **Adults:** (PO): 1 mg 2–3 times/day iniitally Increase to 20 mg/day in 2–4 doses Usual dose 6–15 mg/day	CNS symptoms (dizziness, headache, drowsiness), palpitations, nausea	Caps: 1, 2, 5 mg

Not yet approved or not enough information available for pediatric dosage.

(Continued.)

Drug	Route and Dosage	Toxicity or Side Effects	How Supplied
Propranolol (Inderal) (β-adrenoreceptor blocker)	**Children:** (PO): 2–4 mg/kg/day in 3–4 doses (max 16 mg/kg/day)	Hypotension, syncope	Tab: 10, 20, 40, 60, 80, 90 mg
Reserpine (Serpasil) (depletion of NE store)	**Children:** *For acute hypertension:* (IM): 0.07 mg/kg q8–24h (max 2.5 mg/day) (May be used with hydralazine) (PO): 0.02 mg/kg/day in 2 doses **Adults:** (PO): 0.5 mg/day in 2 doses for 1–2 wk *Maintenance:* 0.1–0.25 mg/day	Hypotension, mental depression, nasal stuffiness	Inj: 2.5 mg/mL Tab: 0.1, 0.25 mg
Tolazoline (Priscoline) (α-adrenoreceptor blocker)	*For neonatal pulmonary hypertension:* (IV): *Loading:* 1–2 mg/kg over 10 min *Maintenance:* 1–2 mg/kg/hr IV infusion *For peripheral vasospastic disease in adults:* (IV): 10–50 mg q4–6h	Hypotension and tachycardia, pulmonary hemorrhage, GI bleeding, arrhythmias	Inj: 25 mg/ml

F. Antiarrhythmic Agents

Amiodarone* (Cordarone) (class III agent)	**Children:** (PO): 5–10 mg/kg/day in 2 doses for 10 days If responsive, 3–5 mg/kg once a day May be reduced to 2.5 mg/kg for 5 of 7 days thereafter **Adults:** (PO): *Loading:* 800–1600 mg/day for 1–3 wk, then reduce to 600–800 mg/day for 1 mo *Maintenance:* 400 mg/day	Nausea/vomiting, corneal microdeposits, hepatotoxicity, progressive dyspnea and cough, worsening of arrhythmias, hypotension and heart block, ataxia, hypo- or hyperthyroidism.	Tab: 200 mg
Bretylium tosylate* (Bretylol) (class III agent)	**Children:** (IV): 5 mg/kg/dose over 8 min, then 10 mg/kg/dose q15–30 min (max 30 mg/kg) *Maintenance:* 5–10 mg/kg/dose q6h **Adults:** (IV): 5–10 mg/kg bolus over 8 min q6h or 1–2 mg/min IV infusion	Hypotension, worsening of arrhythmias, aggravation of digitoxicity, nausea/vomiting	Inj: 50 mg/mL (10 mL amp)

**Not yet approved or not enough information available for pediatric dosage.*

(Continued.)

Drug	Route and Dosage	Toxicity or Side Effects	How Supplied
Disopyramide* (Norpace) (class IA agent)	**Children:** (PO): <1 yr: 10–30 mg/kg/day q6h 1–4 yr: 10–20 mg/kg/day q6h 4–12 yr: 10–15 mg/kg/day q6h 12–18 yr: 6–15 mg/kg/day q6h **Adults:** (PO): *Loading:* 200–300 mg *Maintenance:* 400–800 mg/day q6h (Therapeutic levels: 3–8 μg/mL)	Heart failure/hypotension, anticholinergic effects (urinary retention, dry mouth, constipation), nausea/vomiting, hypoglycemia	Caps: 100, 150 mg
Edrophonium (Tensilon) (acetylcholine-esterase inhibitor)	**Children:** *For SVT:* (IV): 0.1–0.2 mg/kg in single dose (max 10 mg/dose)	Cholinergic crisis (bronchospasm, sedation, nausea/vomiting, diarrhea, lacrimation, involuntary urination or defecation)	Inj: 10 mg/mL (1 mL amp)
Encainide* (Enkaid) (class IC agent)	**Children:** (PO): 2–5 mg/kg/day in 3–4 doses or 60–120 mg/m^2/day in 3–4 doses **Adults:** (PO): 25 mg q8h for 3–5 days Increase to 35–50 mg q8h prn	Worsening of ventricular arrhythmias, CNS symptoms (dizziness, blurred vision, weakness) palpitations, AV block (2nd or 3rd degree), heart failure, hepatotoxicity, hyperglycemia(±)	Caps: 25, 35, 50 mg

Flecainide* (Tambocor) (class IC agent)	**Children:** (IV): 1–2 mg/kg/day in 4 doses **Adults:** (PO): 100 mg q12h for 4 days Increase to 150 mg q12h prn (Max 200 mg q12h)	Worsening of arrhythmias, heart failure, heart block (2nd or 3rd degree), hepatic impairment(±), CNS symptoms (dizziness, visual disturbances, headache)	Tab: 100 mg
Lidocaine (Xylocaine) (class IB agent)	**Children:** (IV): *Loading:* 1 mg/kg/dose q5–10 min prn *Maintenance:* 30 μg/kg/min IV drip (range 20–50 μg/kg/min) **Adults:** (IV): *Loading:* 1 mg/kg/dose q5min *Maintenance:* 1–4 mg/min	Seizure, respiratory depression, CNS symptoms (anxiety, euphoria or drowsiness), arrhythmias, hypotension/shock	Inj: 10 mg/mL (5 mL amp) 20 mg/mL (5, 10 mL amp)
Mexiletine* (Mexitil) (class IB agent)	**Children:** (PO): 4–15 mg/kg/day in 3 doses (with food or antacid) **Adults:** (PO): 200 mg q8h for 2–3 days Increase to 300–400 mg q8h	Nausea/vomiting, CNS symptoms (headache, dizziness, tremor, paresthesia, mood changes), rash, hepatic dysfunction(±)	Caps: 150, 200, 250 mg

**Not yet approved or not enough information available for pediatric dosage.*

(Continued.)

Drug	Route and Dosage	Toxicity or Side Effects	How Supplied
Phenylephrine (Neo-Synephrine)	**Children:** *For SVT:* (IV): 5–10 μg/kg/dose over 20–30 sec	Hypertension, arrhythmias, angina	Inj: 10 mg/mL (1 mL amp)
Phenytoin (Dilantin) (class IB agent)	**Children:** (IV): 2–4 mg/kg/dose over 5–10 min *Followed by:* (PO): 2–5 mg/kg/day in 2–3 doses (Therapeutic levels: 5–18 μg/mL for arrhythmias, 10–20 μg/mL for seizure) **Adults:** (IV): 100 mg q5min (total 500 mg) (PO): 250 mg 4 times for 1 day, 250 mg twice for 2 days, and 300–400 mg/day in 1–4 doses	Rash, Stevens-Johnson syndrome, CNS symptom (ataxia, dysarthria), lupus-like syndrome, blood dyscrasias, peripheral neuropathy, gingival hypertrophy	Inj: 50 mg/mL PO susp: 30, 125 mg/5mL (240 mL) Infatab: 50 mg (chewable) Caps: 30, 100 mg
Procaine amide (Pronestyl) (class IA agent)	**Children:** (IV): *Loading:* 2–3 mg/kg/dose over 5 min repeated q10–30 min prn (max 100 mg) *Maintenance:* 20–80 μg/kg/min (max 2 g/24h) (PO): 40–60 mg/kg/day q3–4h (max 4 g/24h)	Nausea/vomiting, blood dyscrasias, rash, lupus-like syndrome, hypotension, confusion or disorientation	Inj: 100, 500 mg/mL Tab: 250, 375, 500 mg Tab, sustained release: 250, 500, 750, 1,000 mg Caps: 250, 375, 500 mg

	Adults: (IV): *Loading:* 50–100 mg/dose q5min prn *Maintenance:* 1–6 mg/min (PO): 250–500 mg/dose q3–6h (usual dose: 2–4 g/day)		
Propranolol (Inderal) (class II agent [β-adrenergic blocker])	**Children:** (IV): 0.01–0.15 mg/kg/dose over 10 min (max 1 mg/dose) May repeat q6–8h prn (PO): 2–4 mg/kg/day in 4 doses (max 16 mg/kg/day) (Therapeutic levels: 30–100 ng/mL) **Adults:** (IV): 1 mg/dose q5min (max 5 mg) (PO): 40–320 mg/day in 3–4 doses	Hypertension, nausea/vomiting, bronchospasm, hypoglycemia, lethargy or depression, heart block	Inj: 1 mg/mL Tab: 10, 20, 40, 60, 80, 90 mg Caps, sustained release: 120, 160 mg
Quinidine gluconate (class IA agent)	**Children:** (PO): Test for idiosyncracy with 2 mg/kg 10–30 mg/kg/day in 2–3 doses Usual dose 160–660 mg q12h **Adults:** (PO): 25 mg test dose 200–400 mg q4–6h	Nausea/vomiting, ventricular arrhythmias, prolonged QRS, depressed myocardial contractility, blood dyscrasias	Tab, sustained release: 330 mg Inj: 80 mg/mL

(Continued.)

FORMULARY (cont.)

Drug	Route and Dosage	Toxicity or Side Effects	How Supplied
Quinidine sulfate (class IA agent)	**Children:** (PO): Start with 3–6 mg/kg q2–3h for 5 doses May increase to 12 mg/kg q2–3h for 5 doses *Maintenance:* 7–12 mg/kg/day in 4 doses	Same as for quinidine gluconate	Caps: 200, 300 mg Tab: 100, 200, 300 mg Tab, sustained release: 300 mg
Tocainide* (Tonocard) (class IB agent)	**Children:** (PO): 20–40 mg/kg/day in 3 doses **Adults:** (PO): 400 mg q8h May increase to 600 mg q8h Usual dose 400–600 mg q8h	Dizziness/vertigo, nausea/vomiting, blood dyscrasias(±)	Tab: 400 mg
Verapamil (Isoptin, Calan) (class IV agent [Ca channel blocker])	**Children:** (IV): 0–1 yr: 0.1–0.2 mg/kg over 2 min Usual single dose 0.75–2 mg May repeat same dose in 30 min (May be used only when other drugs fail, with extreme caution) 1–15 yr: 0.1–0.3 mg/kg over 2 min. Usual single dose 2–5 mg (max single dose 10 mg). May repeat same dose in 30 min	Hypotension, bradycardia, cardiac depression	Inj: 2.5 mg/mL Tab: 40, 80, 120 mg

	(PO): 3–5 mg/kg/day in 3 doses **Adults:** (IV): 5–10 mg over 2 min May repeat 10 mg in 30 min prn (PO): 240–480 mg/day in 3 doses		
G. Sedatives			
Chloral hydrate (Noctec)	**Children:** *Sedative* (PO,PR): 25 mg/kg/dose q8h *Hypnotic* (PO,PR): 50–75 mg/kg/dose **Adults:** *Sedative* (PO,PR): 250 mg/dose 3 times/day *Hypnotic* (PO,PR): 500–2,000 mg/dose	Mucous membrane irritation (laryngospasm if aspirated), GI irritation, excitement/delirium. (Contraindicated in hepatic and renal impairment)	Syrup: 250, 500 mg/5 mL Supp: 324, 500, 648 mg
Chlorpromazine (Thorazine)	*For sedation or nausea:* **Children** >6 mo: (IM,IV): 0.5 mg/kg/dose q6–8h (PO): 2–3 mg/kg/day q4–6h (PR): 1–2 mg/kg/dose q6–8h **Adults** (IM,IV): 25 mg test dose, then 25–50 mg q3–4h (PO): 10–25 mg q4–6h (PR): 100 mg q6–8h	Hypotension, arrhythmias, 1st-degree AV block, ST-T changes, hepatotoxicity, leukopenia or agranulocytosis	Inj: 25 mg/mL Syrup: 10 mg/5 mL (120 mL) Tab: 10, 25, 50, 100, 200 mg Supp: 25, 100 mg

**Not yet approved or not enough information available for pediatric dosage.*

(Continued.)

FORMULARY (cont.)

Drug	Route and Dosage	Toxicity or Side Effects	How Supplied
Diazepam (Valium)	*For sedation:* **Children:** (IM,IV): 0.1–0.3 mg/kg/dose q2–4h (max 0.6 mg/kg in 8h) (PO): 0.2–0.8 mg/kg/day in 3–4 doses or 1–2.5 mg 3–4 times/day initially and increase prn **Adults:** (IM,IV): 2–10 mg/dose q3–4h prn (PO): 2–10 mg/dose q6–8h prn	Apnea, drowsiness, ataxia, rash	Inj: 5 mg/mL Tab: 2, 5, 10 mg
Hydroxyzine (Vistaril, Atarax)	**Children:** (IM): 1 mg/kg dose q4–6h prn (PO): <6 yr: 50 mg/day in 4 doses >6 yr: 50–100 mg/day in 4 doses **Adults:** (IM): 25–100 mg q4–6h (max 600 mg/day) (PO): 50–100 mg/dose q6h	CNS symptoms (drowsiness, tremor, convulsion), anticholinergic effects (dry mouth, blurred vision, palpitations, hypotension, urinary frequency)	Inj: 25, 50 mg/mL PO susp: 25 mg/5 mL (120 mL) Tab: 10, 25, 50, 100 mg Caps: 25, 50, 100 mg

Ketamine (Ketalar)	**Children:** (IM): 8–12 mg/kg Repeat smaller doses q30min prn (IV): 2 mg/kg/dose Repeat smaller dose q30 min prn	Hypertension/tachycardia, respiratory depression/apnea, CNS symptoms (dreamlike states, confusion, agitation)	Inj: 10, 50, 100 mg/mL
Meperidine (Demerol)	**Children:** (IM,IV,PO): 1–1.5 mg/kg/dose q3–4h prn **Adults:** (IM,IV,PO): 50–100 mg/dose q3–4h prn	CNS or respiratory depression, nausea/vomiting	Inj: 25, 50, 100 mg/mL Tab: 50, 100 mg Syrup: 50 mg/5 mL (16 oz)
Morphine sulfate	**Children:** (SC,IM,IV): 0.1–0.2 mg/kg/dose q2–4h (max 15 mg/dose) **Adults:** (SC,IM,IV): 2.5–20 mg/dose q2–6h prn	CNS depression, respiratory depression, nausea/vomiting, hypotension, bradycardia	Inj: 8, 10, 15, mg/mL
Promethazine (Phenergan)	*For nausea/vomiting:* **Children:** (IM,PO,PR): 0.25–0.5 mg/kg q4–6h prn **Adults:** (IM,PO,PR): 12.5–25 mg q6h prn	CNS stimulation, anticholinergic effects	Inj: 25 & 50 mg/mL Tab: 12.5, 25 & 50 mg Syrup: 6.25 mg/5 mL (4 oz) Supp: 12.5, 25 & 50 mg

(Continued.)

Drug	Route and Dosage	Toxicity or Side Effects	How Supplied
	For sedation/preop: **Children:** (IM): 0.5–1 mg/kg/dose q6h prn **Adults:** (IM,PO,PR): 25–50 mg q4–6h prn		
H. Anticoagulants			
Dicumarol (formerly bishydroxycoumarin)	**Children:** (PO): *Initial dose:* 50–100 mg *Maintenance:* 10–50 mg/day to keep prothrombin time (PT) 1½–2 times control **Adults:** (PO): *Induction:* 200–300 mg *Maintenance:* 25–200 mg/day to keep PT 1½–2 times control	Bleeding (Antidote: vitamin K_1 or fresh-frozen plasma)	Tab: 25, 50 mg
Heparin	**Children:** (IV): *Initial dose:* 50 U/kg *Maintenance:* 100 U/kg q4h (IV drip): 20,000 U/m^2/24h Keep clotting time 2½–3 times control or activated partial thromboplastin time (APTT) 1½–2 times control	Bleeding (Antidote: protamine sulfate)	Inj: 1,000, 5,000, 10,000, 20,000 U/mL

	Adults: (IV): *Initial dose:* 10,000 U *Maintenance:* 5,000–10,000 U q4–6h (IV drip): *Initial dose:* 5,000 U followed by 20,000–40,000 U/day		
Warfarin (Coumadin)	**Children:** (PO): *Initial dose:* 10 mg/day qd for 2–4 days *Maintenance:* 1–5 mg/day once a day Keep PT 1.4–2.5 times control Heparin preferred initially for rapid anticoagulation; warfarin may be started concomitantly with heparin or may be delayed 3–6 days **Adults:** (PO): *Initial dose:* 10 mg/day qd for 2–4 days *Maintenance:* 2–10 mg/day qd	Bleeding (Antidote: vitamin K_1 or fresh-frozen plasma)	Tab: 2, 2.5, 5, 7.5, 10 mg
Vitamin K_1	*Antidote to dicumarol or coumadin:* (PO): 2.5–10 mg in 1 dose for correction of excessive PT from dicumarol or warfarin overdose		Tab: 5 mg

(Continued.)

Drug	Route and Dosage	Toxicity or Side Effects	How Supplied
Protamine sulfate	*Antidote to heparin overdose:* (IV): Slow IV infusion of no more than 50 mg in any 10 min (each 1 mg protamine neutralizes approx 100 U heparin)	Coagulation problem	Inj: 10 mg/mL
I. Lipid and Cholesterol Lowering Agents			
Cholestyramine (Questran)	**Children:** (PO): 250–1,500 mg/kg/day in 2–4 doses **Adults:** (PO): 9 g (1 packet or 1 scoopful) 1–6 times/day (mix with 2–6 oz water or other fluid)	Constipation/other GI symptoms, hyperchloremic acidosis, bleeding	Packet: 9 g (4 g anhydrous cholestyramine resin)
Colestipol* (Colestid)	**Children:** (PO): 300–1,500 mg/day in 2–4 doses **Adults:** (PO): 15–30 g/day in 2–4 doses (mix with 3–6 oz water or other fluid)	Constipation/other GI symptoms (abdominal distention, flatulence, nausea/vomiting, diarrhea), rarely rash, muscle and joint pain, headache, dizziness	Packet: 5 g

Clofibrate* (Atromid-S)	**Children:** (PO): 0.5–1.5 mg/day in 2–3 doses **Adults:** (PO): 2 g/day in 2–3 doses	Nausea/other GI symptoms (vomiting, diarrhea, flatulence), headache, dizziness, fatigue, rash, blood dyscrasias, myalgia/arthralgia, hepatic dysfunction	Caps: 500 mg
Nicotinic acid	**Children:** (PO): 25–75 mg/kg/day in 2–3 doses, taken with meals	Hepatic dysfunction, nausea/vomiting, flushing	Tab: 100, 500, 1,000 mg
J. Miscellaneous			
Allopurinol (Zyloprim) (uric acid biosynthesis inhibitor)	(PO): 10 mg/kg/day in 4 doses (Max 600 mg/day) After 2 days titrate dose according to serum uric acid	Rash, urticaria, fever, GI irritation, leukocytosis/eosinophilia, hepatotoxicity, neuritis	Tab: 100, 300 mg
Indomethacin (Indocin)	*For PDA closure in premature infants:* (IV): 0.2 mg/kg, then 0.1–0.2 mg/kg, up to 2 doses, q12h prn (total up to 3 doses)	GI or other bleeding, GI disturbances, renal impairment, electrolyte disturbances (↓Na, ↑K)	Vial: 1 mg

Not yet approved or not enough information available for pediatric dosage.

(Continued.)

FORMULARY (cont.).

Drug	Route and Dosage	Toxicity or Side Effects	How Supplied
Naloxone (Narcan)	**Children:** (IM, IV): 5–10 μg/kg/dose q2–3 min for 1–3 doses prn (may need 5–10 doses) **Adults:** (IM, IV): 0.4–2 mg/dose q2–3 min for 1–3 doses prn	Allergy, ventricular arrhythmias, pulmonary edema(±).	Inj: 0.4 mg/mL 0.02 mg/mL (for neonate)
Potassium chloride	*For diuretic therapy:* (PO): 1–2 mEq/kg/day in 3–4 doses or 0.8–1.5 mL 10% sol/kg/day or 0.4–0.7 mL 20% sol/kg/day	GI disturbances, ulcerations, hyperkalemia	10% sol: 1.3 mEq/mL 20% sol: 2.7 mEq/mL
Potassium gluconate (Kaon)	*For diuretic therapy:* (PO): 1–2 mEq/kg/day in 3–4 doses or 0.8–1.5 mL/kg/day	Same as for potassium chloride	Elixir: 1.3 mEq/mL
Potassium triplex (acetate-bicarbonate-citrate)	*For diuretic therapy:* (PO): 1–2 mEq/kg/day in 3–4 doses or 0.3–0.6 mL/kg/day	Same as for potassium chloride	PO sol: 3 mEq/mL

Prostaglandin E_1 (Prostin VR, Alprostadil)	*For patency of ductus arteriosus:* (IV): Begin infusion at 0.05–0.1 μg/kg/min When desired effects achieved, reduce to 0.05, 0.025, and 0.01 μg/kg/min If unresponsive, dose may be increased to 0.4 μg/kg/min	Apnea, flushing, brady/tachycardia, hypotension, fever	Amp: 500 μg/mL
Sodium polystyrene (Kayexalate)	*For hyperkalemia* (slowly effective, taking hours to days): **Children:** (PO,NG): 1 g/kg/dose q6h (PR): 1 g/kg/dose q2–6h **Adults:** (PO,NG,PR): 15 g (4 level tsp) 1–4 times/day	(Cation exchange resin with practical exchange rates of 1 mEq K/1 g resin) NOTE: delivers 1 mEq Na for each mEq K removed Nausea/vomiting, constipation, severe hypokalemia (monitor serum K, ECG, muscle weakness, confusion), hypocalcemia/hypernatremia (edema)	Powder: 454 g/lb Susp: 15 g/60 mL

APPENDIX

FIG A–1.
A and **B,** antibiotic prophylaxis against bacterial endocarditis, as recommended by the American Heart Association. (Used by permission.)

Name: ____________________

needs protection from

BACTERIAL ENDOCARDITIS

because of an existing

HEART CONDITION

Diagnosis: ____________________

Prescribed by: ____________________

Date: ____________________

For Dental Procedures and Surgery of the Upper Respiratory Tract

1. For most patients: **Oral Penicillin**	**Adults:** 2.0 g of penicillin V one hour prior to procedure and then 1.0 g six hours after initial dose. **Children less than 60 pounds:** 1.0 g of penicillin V one hour prior to procedure and then 500 mg six hours after initial dose.
2. For those allergic to penicillin (may also be selected for those receiving oral penicillin as continuous rheumatic fever prophylaxis): **Erythromycin**	**Adults:** 1.0 g orally one hour prior to procedure and then 500 mg six hours after initial dose. **Children:** 20 mg/kg orally one hour prior to procedure and then 10 mg/kg six hours after initial dose.
3. For those patients at higher risk of infective endocarditis (especially those with prosthetic heart valves) who are not allergic to penicillin: **Ampicillin** plus **Gentamicin**	**Adults:** Ampicillin 1.0-2.0 g plus gentamicin 1.5 mg/kg IM or IV, both given 30 minutes before procedure; then penicillin V 1.0 g (500 mg for children under 60 lb) orally six hours after initial dose. **Children:** Timing of doses is same as for adults. Dosages are ampicillin 50 mg/kg and gentamicin 2.0 mg/kg.
4. For higher risk patients (especially those with prosthetic heart valves) who are allergic to penicillin: **Vancomycin**	**Adults:** Vancomycin 1 g IV over 60 minutes, begun 60 minutes before procedure; no repeat dose is necessary. **Children:** Vancomycin 20 mg/kg IV over 60 minutes, begun 60 minutes before procedure; no repeat dose is necessary.

For Gastrointestinal and Genitourinary Tract Surgery and Instrumentation	
1. For most patients: **Ampicillin** plus **Gentamicin**	**Adults**: 2.0 g ampicillin IM or IV plus gentamicin 1.5 mg/kg IM or IV given 30 minutes before procedure. May repeat once eight hours later. **Children**: Same timing of medications as adult schedule. Dosages are ampicillin 50 mg/kg and gentamicin 2.0 mg/kg.
2. For patients allergic to penicillin: **Vancomycin** plus **Gentamicin**	**Adults**: 1.0 g vancomycin IV given over 60 minutes plus 1.5 mg/kg gentamicin IM or IV, each given 60 minutes before procedure. Doses may be repeated once 8-12 hours later. **Children**: Timing as above. Doses are vancomycin 20 mg/kg and gentamicin 2.0 mg/kg.
3. Oral regimen for minor or repetitive procedures in low-risk patients: **Amoxicillin**	**Adults**: 3.0 g amoxicillin one hour before procedure and 1.5 g six hours after initial dose. **Children**: Same timing of doses: 50 mg/kg initial dose and 25 mg/kg follow-up dose.

Note: In patients with compromised renal function, it may be necessary to modify or omit the second dose of antibiotics. Intramuscular injections may be contraindicated in patients receiving anticoagulants. Children's doses should not exceed adult doses.

FIG A–1 (cont.)

Adapted from A Statement for Health Professionals by the Committee on Rheumatic Fever and Infective Endocarditis: Prevention of Bacterial Endocarditis. *Circulation* 1984; 70:1123A-1127A (also excerpted in *J Am Dent Assoc* 1985;110:98-100).

Please refer to these joint American Heart Association–American Dental Association recommendations for more complete information as to which patients and which procedures require prophylaxis.

American Heart Association

National Center
7320 Greenville Avenue
Dallas, Texas 75231

78-004-D (CP)
85-88-1.510MM
3-89-500M
85 01 24 D

Accepted
COUNCIL ON DENTAL THERAPEUTICS
AMERICAN DENTAL ASSOCIATION

The Council on Dental Therapeutics of the American Dental Association has approved this statement as it relates to dentistry.

FIG A–1 (cont.)

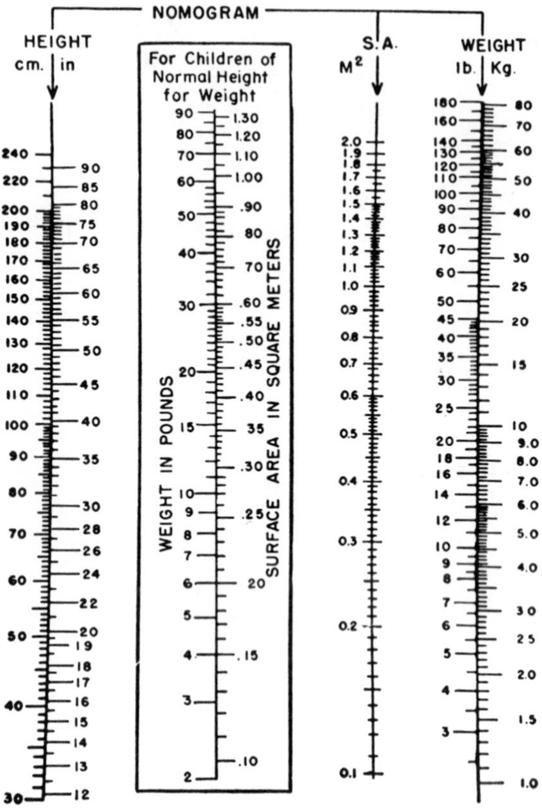

FIG A–2.
Body surface nomogram.

TABLE A–1.

Normal M-Mode Echocardiographic Dimensions (mm) by Weight (lb): Mean (Range)*

	Weight (lb)					
	0–25	26–50	51–75	76–100	101–125	126–200
RV dimension	9 (3–15)	10 (4–15)	11 (7–18)	12 (7–16)	13 (8–17)	13 (12–17)
LV dimension	24 (13–32)	34 (24–38)	38 (33–45)	41 (35–47)	43 (37–49)	49 (44–52)
LV free wall (or septum)	5 (4–6)	6 (5–7)	7 (6–7)	7 (7–8)	7 (7–8)	8 (7–8)
LA dimension	17 (7–23)	22 (17–27)	23 (19–28)	24 (20–30)	27 (21–30)	28 (21–37)
Aortic root	13 (7–17)	17 (13–22)	20 (17–23)	22 (19–27)	23 (17–27)	24 (22–28)

**Adapted from Feigenbaum H: Echocardiography*, ed 4. Philadelphia, Lea & Febiger, 1986.

TABLE A–2.

Other Normal M-Mode Echo Values: Mean (95% CI)

LA/Ao ratio:	1.1 (0.7–1.6)
IVS/LVPW ratio:	1.1 (0.8–1.5)
FS = (LVDD – LVSD)/LVDD:	0.36 (0.28–0.44)
EF = $(LVDD)^3 - (LVSD)^3$ $/(LVDD)^3 \times 100$:	74% (64%–83%)
LPEP/LVET:	0.35 (0.30–0.39)
RPEP/RVET:	0.24 (0.16–0.30)

LA = left atrium, Ao = aorta, IVS = interventricular septum, LVPW = left ventricular posterior wall, FS = fractional shortening, EF = ejection fraction, LVDD = left ventricular diastolic dimension, LVSD = left ventricular systolic dimension, L(R)PEP = left (right) preejection period, LV(RV)ET = left (right) ventricular ejection time.

TABLE A–3.

Normal M-Mode Echo Measurements (mm): Mean (95% prediction interval)*†

BW(kg)	3	5	8	10	15	20	25	30	40	50	60	70
BSA (m^2)	0.24	0.34	0.45	0.52	0.68	0.82	0.94	1.06	1.27	1.47	1.65	1.82
IVS	4.5 (3.5–5)	4.5 (4–5.5)	5 (4.5–6)	5.5 (4.5–6.5)	6 (5–7)	7 (5.5–8.5)	7 (5.5–9)	7.5 (6–9)	8.5 (6.5–10)	8.5 (7–10)	9 (8–10.5)	9.5 (7.5–11)
LVPW	4 (3.5–5)	4.5 (4–5)	5 (4–6)	5 (4.5–6)	6 (5–7)	6.5 (5.5–8)	7 (6–8)	7 (6–8.5)	8 (6.5–9)	8.5 (7–9.5)	8.5 (7.5–10)	9 (7.5–11)
AO	12 (10–14)	13 (11–16)	15 (12–17)	16 (13–18)	18 (15–22)	19 (16–23)	21 (17–24)	22 (18–26)	23 (19–27)	25 (20–29)	26 (21–30)	27 (23–32)
LA	18 (15–21)	20 (16–23)	21 (17–25)	22 (18–26)	25 (21–29)	27 (22–32)	28 (23–33)	30 (24–35)	32 (26–37)	33 (27–38)	34 (28–41)	36 (29–42)
LVDD	21 (18–23)	25 (22–27)	28 (24–31)	29 (25–32)	33 (29–36)	35 (31–39)	37 (33–41)	39 (34–43)	42 (37–47)	44 (39–49)	46 (41–51)	48 (42–53)
LVSD	14 (12–17)	16 (13–19)	17 (14–21)	18 (15–22)	21 (17–24)	23 (18–27)	24 (19–28)	25 (21–29)	27 (22–32)	28 (23–33)	29 (24–34)	31 (25–36)

**Adapted from data presented in graphic form by Henry WL, Ware J, Gardin JM, et al: Circulation 1987; 57:278–285.*

†Values rounded off to the nearest 0.5 mm for IVS and LVPW and to the nearest 1.0 mm all other measurements.

AO = aorta, IVS = interventricular septum, LA = left atrium, LVDD = left ventricular diastolic dimension, LVPW = left ventricular posterior wall, LVSD = left ventricular systolic dimension.

TABLE A–4.

Dimensions of Aorta and Pulmonary Arteries by 2D Echo*†

Echo Views	BSA (m^2)	0.25	0.3	0.4	0.5
	BW(kg)	3	4	7	10
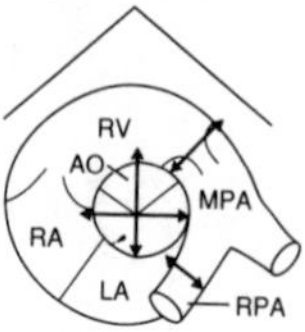	Ascending aorta	10 (7–13)	11 (7.5–15)	13 (9–16)	14 (10–18)
	MPA	9 (5–12)	10 (6–13)	11 (7–14)	12 (8–16)
	RPA	5.5 (3.5–8)	6 (4–8.5)	6.5 (4.5–9)	7.5 (5–10)
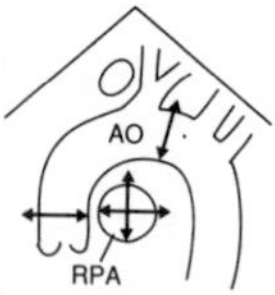	Ascending aorta	7.5 (4–10)	8 (4.5–11)	9 (6–12)	10 (6.5–13)
	Transverse aorta	6 (4–8.5)	7 (4.5–9)	8 (5.5–11)	9 (6.5–11)
	RPA	6 (4–8)	6.5 (4.5–9)	7.5 (5–10)	8.5 (6–11)
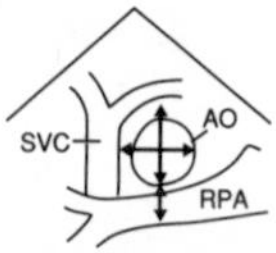	Transverse aorta	9 (6–11)	10 (7–12.5)	11 (8–14)	12 (9.5–15)
	RPA	6 (4–8)	6.5 (4.5–9)	7 (5–10)	8 (6–10)

**Adapted from data presented in graphic form by Snider AR, Enderlein MA, Teitel DF, et al: Am J Cardiol* 1984; 53:218–224.

†Values rounded off to nearest 0.5 mm for measurements <10 mm and to nearest 1.0 mm for measurements ≥10 mm. Figures in pa-

0.6	0.7	0.8	0.9	1.0	1.2	1.4
13	16	19	23	28	37	46
15 (11–19)	16 (12–20)	17 (12–21)	17 (13–22)	18 (14–23)	20 (15–25)	22 (16–27)
13 (9–17)	14 (9–18)	15 (11–19)	15 (11–20)	16 (12–21)	17 (13–23)	19 (14–24)
8 (5.5–10)	8.5 (6–11)	9 (7–11)	9 (7–12)	10 (7–12)	10 (8–14)	11 (8–15)
11 (7.5–14)	12 (8.5–15)	12 (9–16)	13 (9.5–13)	14 (11–18)	15 (12–19)	17 (14–21)
10 (7.5–12)	11 (8–13)	11 (8.5–14)	12 (9.5–15)	13 (10–16)	14 (11–17)	15 (12–18)
9 (6.5–11)	9.5 (7–12)	10 (8–13)	11 (9–14)	12 (9–15)	13 (10–16)	14 (11–17)
13 (10.5–16)	14 (11–17)	15 (13–18)	16 (13–20)	17 (14–20)	19 (15–22)	20 (17–24)
9 (6.5–11)	9.5 (7.5–11)	10 (8–12)	11 (9–13)	11 (9–14)	12 (10–15)	13 (11–16)

rentheses are tolerance limits weighted for BSA for prediction of normal values for 80% of future population with 50% confidence. Measurements are made at end-diastolic (Q wave) using leading-edge technique.

TABLE A–5.

Mitral and Tricuspid Valve Annulus Diameter by 2D Echo: Mean (95% CI)*†

BSA (m^2)	0.2	0.25	0.3	0.4	0.5	0.6	0.7	0.8	0.9	1.0	1.2	1.4
BW (kg)	2	3	4	7	10	13	16	19	23	28	37	46
Mitral valve	10	12	13	16	18	19	21	22	23	24	25	26
(PL)	(7–13)	(9–15)	(10–16)	(13–19)	(15–21)	(16–23)	(18–24)	(18–26)	(19–26)	(20–27)	(22–28)	(23–30)
Mitral valve	12	15	17	20	23	25	27	29	31	32	35	36
(A4C, S4C)‡	(7–17)	(10–20)	(12–22)	(16–25)	(18–28)	(20–31)	(22–32)	(23–35)	(25–36)	(26–37)	(28–40)	(31–42)
Tricuspid valve	12	15	17	21	23	26	27	29	31	32	34	36
(A4C, S4C)‡	(8–17)	(10–19)	(12–22)	(16–26)	(18–29)	(20–31)	(22–33)	(23–36)	(24–37)	(25–38)	(27–42)	(28–44)

**Adapted from data presented in graphic form by King DH, Smith EO, Huhta JC, et al:* Am J Cardiol *1985; 55:787–789.*
†Measurements made at onset of R wave on ECG, using inner edge–to–inner edge method.
‡Measurements greater of two projections; A4C and S4C.
A4C = apical four-chamber view; S4C = subcostal four-chamber view; PL = parasternal long-axis view.

TABLE A–6.

Normal Doppler Velocities in Children (cm/sec)

Site	Mean (range)	Site	Mean (range)
SVC	51 (28–80)	LA (peak)	58 (45–80)
RA (peak)	47 (38–74)	LV inflow	78 (44–128)
RV Inflow	62 (41–84)	Asc. aorta	97 (60–154)
MPA	76 (50–105)	Desc. aorta	102 (70–160)

From Goldberg SJ, Allen HD, Marx GR, et al: Doppler Echocardiography. *Philadelphia, Lea & Febiger, 1985, pp 34–54.*

TABLE A–7.

Doppler Echocardiographic Formulas

1. Pressure gradient (ΔP) = $4(V_2^2 - V_1^2)$
   If $V_1 < 1$ m/sec, $\Delta P = 4(V_{max})^2$
2. Flow (mL/min) = $\dfrac{\text{Mean velocity (cm/sec)} \times \text{Flow area (cm}^2\text{)} \times 60 \text{ (sec/min)}}{\text{Cosine of intercept angle*}}$

   *Cos θ: 0° = 1.00; 10° = 0.98; 20° = 0.94; 30° = 0.87;
   40° = 0.77; 50° = 0.64.
3. Aortic (pulmonary) valve area (cm²) = $\dfrac{SV}{(0.9)(V_{max})(SEP)}$

   where SV = stroke volume; SEP = systolic ejection period.
4. Mitral valve area (cm²) = $\dfrac{220}{\text{Pressure half-time (sec)}}$

TABLE A–8.

Oxygen Consumption per Body Surface Area [(mL/min)/m^2] by Sex, Age and Heart Rate

Age (yr)	Heart Rate (bpm) 50	60	70	80	90	100	110	120	130	140	150	160	170
Male patients													
3				155	159	163	167	171	175	178	182	186	190
4			149	152	156	160	163	168	171	175	179	182	186
6		141	144	148	151	155	159	162	167	171	174	178	181
8		136	141	145	148	152	156	159	163	167	171	175	178
10	130	134	139	142	146	149	153	157	160	165	169	172	176
12	128	132	136	140	144	147	151	155	158	162	167	170	174
14	127	130	134	137	142	146	149	153	157	160	165	169	172
16	125	129	132	136	141	144	148	152	155	159	162	167	
18	124	127	131	135	139	143	147	150	154	157	161	166	
20	123	126	130	134	137	142	145	149	153	156	160	165	
25	120	124	127	131	135	139	143	147	150	154	157		
30	118	122	125	129	133	136	141	145	148	152	155		
35	116	120	124	127	131	135	139	143	147	150			
40	115	119	122	126	130	133	137	141	145	149			

Female patients													
3				150	153	157	161	165	169	172	176	180	183
4			141	145	149	152	156	159	163	168	171	175	179
6		130	134	137	142	146	149	153	156	160	165	168	172
8		125	129	133	136	141	144	148	152	155	159	163	167
10	118	122	125	129	133	136	141	144	148	152	155	159	163
12	115	119	122	126	130	133	137	141	145	149	152	156	160
14	112	116	120	123	127	131	134	133	143	146	150	153	157
16	109	114	118	121	125	128	132	136	140	144	148	151	
18	107	111	116	119	123	127	130	134	137	142	146	149	
20	106	109	114	118	121	125	128	132	136	140	144	148	
25	102	106	109	114	118	121	125	128	132	136	140		
30	99	103	106	110	115	118	122	125	129	133	136		
35	97	100	104	107	111	116	119	123	127	130			
50	94	98	102	105	109	112	117	121	124	128			

From LaFarge CG, Miettinen, OS: Cardiovasc Res 1970; 4:23. Used by permission.

SUGGESTED READINGS

1. Adams FH, Emmanouilides GC, Riemenschneider TA: *Moss' Heart Disease in Infants, Children, and Adolescents,* ed 4, Baltimore, Williams & Wilkins Co, 1989.
2. Anthony CL, Arnon RG: *Pediatric Cardiology,* rev ed. New Hyde Park, NY, Medical Examination Publishing Co, 1983.
3. Feigenbaum H: *Echocardiography,* ed. 4. Philadelphia, Lea & Febiger, 1986.
4. Keith JD, Rowe RD, Vlad P: *Heart Disease in Infancy and Childhood,* ed 3. New York, Macmillan Publishing Co, 1978.
5. Kirklin JW, Barratt-Boyes BG: *Cardiac Surgery,* New York, John Wiley & Sons, 1986.
6. Park MK, *Pediatric Cardiology for Practitioners,* ed 2. Chicago, Year Book Medical Publishers, 1988.
7. Park MK, Guntheroth WG: *How to Read Pediatric ECGs,* ed 2. Chicago, Year Book Medical Publishers, 1987.
8. Snider AR, Serwer GA: *Echocardiography in Pediatric Heart Disease.* Chicago, Year Book Medical Publishers, 1990.
9. Rudolph AM: *Congenital Diseases of the Heart,* Chicago, Year Book Medical Publishers, 1974.

Index

C

E

F

G

H

P

S

T

U

V